Vestibular Migraine

Vestibular Migraine

A comprehensive patient guide

Mark Knoblauch PhD

Kiremma Press

Houston, TX

Printed in the United States of America

Disclaimer: **This book is not intended and must not be used as a substitute for the medical advice of licensed medical professionals. The reader should regularly consult his or her physician in any matter relating to his/her health and particularly with respect to any symptoms that may require diagnosis of a medical attention.**

www.authorMK.com

ISBN: 978-1-7320674-5-5

This book quickly turned from what I felt was a work of necessity into a work of discovery. Through researching the material for this book, I soon learned of the vast control that vestibular migraine can wield over its sufferers.

Therefore, to all who have to suffer through every day with the incapacitating effects of vestibular migraine, this book is dedicated to you.

Table of Contents

Introduction

FOR ANYONE WHO HAS HAD VERTIGO, they know the misery associated with the constant spinning and unsteadiness. Likewise, migraine sufferers are all too familiar with the pain and debilitation that severe headaches can bring. Combine vertigo with headache into what is known as a *vestibular migraine* and the effects can be overwhelming, frustrating, and often inconvenient all at once. Other times the symptoms can just be flat-out annoying. If you have purchased this book, it's likely that you or someone close to you has been dealing with vestibular migraine at some level, whether that be severe and incapacitating or just bothersome. The random vertigo attacks that are often tied in with headaches can tend to encompass all aspects of your daily life, from your sleep to your work to your most intimate moments. And what can be particularly frustrating is that you often don't 'look' sick; rather, you seem quite normal during those times that friends, family, or colleagues see you. That's because those individuals don't see you during your worst – those times when you find a quiet secluded place to let your attacks run their course, safe from the view of others. This practice of having your attacks in seclusion often leaves those around you empathetic towards your plight but at the same time not able to fully understand the frustration and often anger you are experiencing, not to mention the uncontrollable effects of the attacks that you experience. This anger can often be amplified when you find that medical providers can't figure out what is going on, at times even arriving at a final diagnosis of *anxiety* and telling you to just try to relax. This in turn makes you feel as though people think it's 'all in your head'. And while it is true from a physiological standpoint that vestibular migraine is indeed all 'in your head', it is in no way limited to being just a psychological condition. The effects can become infuriating to say the least.

Despite its prevalence within the population, the cause as well as effective treatment for vestibular migraine eludes us. In the world of medicine though, vestibular migraine is relatively new as a recognized condition; just a couple decades ago there was no established medical diagnosis and as a result there was little devoted treatment. Evidence of the relatively 'recent' interest in vestibular migraine can be found in the evidence showing that since 1990, the number of articles that discuss vertigo and headache has effectively doubled every five years[1]. As the year 2000 turned, a growing shift in awareness began to occur toward vestibular migraine, which in turn drew attention to the specific set of symptoms involved. This focus on specific symptoms then allowed medical professionals to start to hone in on these symptoms as a true and recognized medical condition, thereby encouraging the development of directed treatments.

In the past 20 years since vestibular migraine research began to gain steam, medicine and science have learned a lot about the inner ear. We have been able to pinpoint the cause of many conditions of the inner ear, including some which are much less common than vestibular migraine. However, people are still significantly affected by vestibular migraine, which means we haven't progressed as far as we might want. But as you will read in this book, vestibular migraine is a tricky beast. It doesn't follow a consistent pattern from one patient to the next. It often mimics other medical conditions. And despite its name, it doesn't always elicit a headache or vestibular-related event. In light of these complications, the need for further research is certainly warranted. This also means that funding, technology, and likely even pharmaceutical treatments must continue to be generated. And as current research continues, we are beginning to learn that the factors involved in vestibular migraine may be more complex than we first thought, likely resulting not from a single issue or event but rather a complex assortment of interactions between our ear, brain, and head that emerge as a single condition. Yet even though medicine has been successful at curing many diseases and conditions, vestibular migraine's cure still escapes us.

While a cure remains to be found for vestibular migraine, that is not to say that patients are left unable to defend themselves from its onslaught. Treatments have been shown to be effective for many individuals even though other sufferers may have no effect from an identical treatment. In the world of conditions that have no cure, patients are often willing to try anything, even experimenting on their own in order to try to get some sort of relief from what they're experiencing. But there is a bright spot in all of this – the more things we try as treatment for vestibular migraine, the more things we learn specific to what works and what doesn't work. And as we discover new treatments that become effective, we at the same time can begin to hone in on *why* those treatments work – what they are doing within the body and what tissues they are targeting. Every small bit of information that we learn helps add one more piece to the puzzle of finding a cure for vestibular migraine. The more we know, the more ammunition we have to fight this miserable disease.

Similarly, this book is intended to serve as your own small bit of ammunition against vestibular migraine. It was conceived and designed to serve as a resource to help you learn more about this frustrating condition and perhaps even provide you options to deal with your own symptoms. Because vestibular migraine is thought to be involved with those structures in the ear responsible for assisting us with balance and detection of motion, we will start this book off by reviewing the relevant anatomy of the inner ear. We'll then take a look at the second component of vestibular migraine and outline what a traditional migraine is as well as how it can be treated. Next we'll review relevant recent research about vestibular migraine including the variety of suspected causes, demographics, prevalence, and symptoms. By understanding these foundational aspects of vestibular migraine you can better appreciate just how complex the condition is, in turn helping you to understand why a cure remains so elusive. We'll also focus on how vestibular migraine affects children specifically, including how the disease differs from vestibular migraine in adults. Next, we'll look at the diagnostic criteria associated with vestibular migraine, focusing on what conditions and symptoms must be present in order to establish a diagnosis of vestibular migraine.

Because I have had a long history with vestibular conditions as well as ongoing headaches, I'll then outline for you my own experience with these symptoms – from when I first woke up extremely dizzy to my days of perpetual headaches. We'll then look at treatments associated with vestibular migraine, including the pharmaceutical options that are available for sufferers. Because vertigo and headache are both common symptoms of many medical ailments, we'll outline a few of the most common associated conditions that can mimic what vestibular migraine sufferers experience. Finally, we'll close the book out with a look at how vestibular migraine affects a patient's quality of life, focusing on not only the reported effects of vestibular migraine but also taking a look at this condition from a patient's perspective.

If you or someone you know has been newly diagnosed with – or is living with – vestibular migraine, this book has been written for you. You will likely have a series of initial frustrations in dealing with this disorder just like so many other sufferers have encountered, and this book is written to help get you through those initial stages and help you work with your medical professional to manage your vestibular migraine over time. My hope is that this book will not only make you a better-informed vestibular migraine patient but will also help you understand how to maintain a normal lifestyle despite having the sometimes-debilitating attacks that can seem to come out of nowhere.

If you are a vestibular migraine patient, don't give up hope. There are many treatment options out there, and keep in mind that the initial stages of dealing with vestibular migraine can be the worst. Over time you'll likely recognize triggers that can help reduce both the severity and frequency of attacks, not to mention a potential reduction in doctor visits and testing procedures that you will be put through in order to establish what is going on. Always remember that the right treatments and avoidance of triggers can make an amazing difference in your dealings with vestibular migraine, with the hope of ultimately returning you to that quality of life that existed prior to your having vestibular migraine. Now, let's start our journey together with this book, a first step towards getting you on your path to taking control of your vestibular migraine.

Chapter 1: Anatomy of the Ear

WHILE MIGRAINES TEND TO BE associated with some aspect of the brain, vestibular migraines often involve a component of severe unsteadiness and vertigo than can often compound the effects of the concurrent migraine. In many cases, symptoms such as vertigo, dizziness, or unsteadiness originate within the structures of the inner ear. Therefore, we'll now take a look at the general anatomy and physiology of those inner ear structures that play a role in vertigo as well as imbalance and unsteadiness. To understand how these symptoms occur we have to first outline how the structures that are capable of generating vertigo actually work. Therefore, this chapter is dedicated to detailing the intricacies of the inner ear, particularly those structures that are responsible for detecting motion. In describing the structure and function of the vestibular system of the inner ear, it provides a foundation to help understand how vertigo and unsteadiness are generated within the body.

We tend to think of our ear as that funny flap of skin that exists on the sides of our head. However, the true extent of our ear is much more than that. In fact, the *pinna* – the part of the ear that we can see – is actually the least involved structure of all, as it has minimal influence on our ability to detect sound or movement. The truly functional parts of our ears exist deep inside of our skulls in an area called the *inner ear*, a portion of our skull that is comprised of very delicate structures. Because of their delicate nature, these sensitive structures within our inner ear are subject to damage due to causes such trauma, such as might occur when getting hit in the head with a ball, or disease, as could occur due to a serious ear infection. Injury to the structures of the ear can cause not only diminished hearing or deafness, but also a variety of vestibular-related problems such as dizziness, unsteadiness, or vertigo.

Although we know that the inner ear is involved in hearing and equilibrium, it is important to understand that the ear merely *detects* sound and motion – it does not 'interpret' sound nor process any motion that we make. Rather, processing of sound is a function of our brain that occurs in response to input received from those sensors deep within our ear structure. Because the brain and portions of the inner ear work together to detect and process movement, the inner ear is often noted as the 'peripheral vestibular organ' while areas specific to the brain (e.g. cerebellum, brain stem) are considered the 'central' vestibular organs.

Most often, vestibular conditions are associated with structures of the ear. For example, benign paroxysmal positional vertigo (BPPV) is a vertigo-inducing condition that results when small calcium crystals within the inner ear become dislodged and influence the motion sensors of the inner ear. Vestibular migraine, however, is not as clearly defined in terms of origins or affected structures. However, as vertigo is a major component of vestibular migraine (the word 'vestibular' itself relates to an area of the inner ear), it's pertinent to take time to look at just what all is involved in the structure and function of the inner ear. This will help set a foundation for you as to how balance and equilibrium are detected by the body, both of which can be significantly affected by vestibular migraine. Keep in mind that the anatomy and physiology of the inner ear thought to be involved with vestibular migraine is likely related largely to those structures responsible for *detecting* motion. The interpretation and processing of that detected motion is performed deep within the brain.

One point of clarification must be made specific to the anatomy involved with vestibular migraine. There's no doubt that the brain is highly involved in vestibular migraine. However, unlike the inner ear with its clearly defined structures, we know much less about the specific areas of the brain, particularly how these areas influence vestibular migraine. Therefore, we won't be outlining the different areas of the brain in this chapter but will instead focus on those structures within the ear that play a major role in our ability to detect motion.

Outer ear

The outer ear is the portion of the ear that we can see (Figure 1.1). This includes the large pinna as well as the ear canal that leads to the eardrum. The function of the outer ear is largely limited to funneling sound into the eardrum, and as it is located well away from the inner ear structures that are involved with vestibular migraine, the outer ear is not considered to have any involvement with vestibular migraine.

Middle ear

The middle ear is the air-filled portion of the ear located behind the eardrum and housed within the temporal bone (Figure 1.1). This portion of the ear holds the three

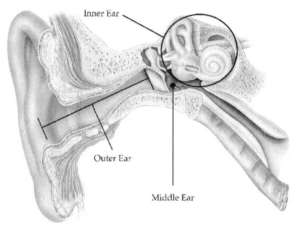

Figure 1.1. The three sections of the ear include the outer ear, middle ear, and inner ear. Issues involved with vestibular migraine are suspected to originate within the labyrinth portion of the inner ear

small bones – the malleus, stapes, and incus – that transfer sound from the eardrum to the inner ear. The most you will likely deal with the middle ear is when you suffer the effects of an ear infection. As the middle ear is really nothing more than a space within the temporal bone, it has no specific involvement with vestibular migraine.

Inner ear

The inner ear is responsible for both detecting and converting sound waves to neural impulses, and also plays a role in the perception and interpretation of body positioning. The inner ear is comprised of an array of highly sensitive structures, which also makes the inner ear somewhat susceptible to injury. Because of the high level of involvement of the inner ear structures in detecting sound and motion, the inner ear has been called one of the most intensively studied areas of vertebrate anatomy and physiology[2]. Despite its small size, intricate structure, and dual responsibility for handling detection of both sound and motion, damage to the sensitive components of the inner ear can affect hearing as well as equilibrium, and even minor disruptive events can trigger several symptoms such as motion sickness, vertigo or nausea.

There are two main areas that make up the inner ear – the cochlea and the vestibular system. Together, these two structures make up what is known as the *labyrinth*. Despite what you often see in images of the inner ear, the labyrinth organs are not free-standing organs; rather, they are actually tunnels that exist deep within the temporal bone (Figure 1.2). These tunnels contain membranes that serve to maintain the unique fluid (i.e. 'endolymph') housed within the labyrinth. As we will discuss, it is the movement of this fluid within the vestibular system that provides much of our ability to detect certain motions of the head.

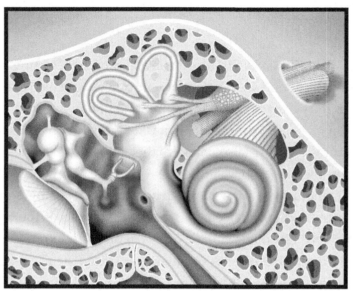

Figure 1.2. The cochlea and vestibular system are housed within the matrix of the temporal bone. Though actually formed by the bone, the labyrinth organs are lined with membranes that house the endolymph fluid of the inner ear.

Vestibular system

The vestibular system of the inner ear serves to detect body motion as well as head position (Figure 1.3). It is generally accepted that the structures making up the vestibular organs are involved in vestibular migraine, so we will outline in detail the relevant anatomy of the vestibular organs.

Five independent structures are involved in our ability to detect motion. The first two structures are housed within the vestibule, a 3-5mm wide organ located between the cochlea and semicircular canals. The vestibule holds the two structures - the saccule and the utricle – responsible for detecting motion that occurs in a linear plane (i.e. forward/backward, up/down, side-to-side). Activities such as running, walking, standing up, or even riding in an elevator are detected by the saccule and the utricle, both of which contain small calcium-based crystals that provide

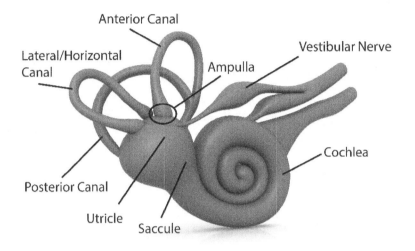

Figure 1.3. The labyrinth system is a specialized structure consisting of organs used for detection of sound as well as registering head motion.

feedback about the direction of motion. Because the saccule and utricle house these small crystals known as *otoliths*, the utricle and saccule are known as the "otolith organs". In addition to these two structures, the remainder of the vestibular portion of the inner ear is comprised of three 'tubes' called semicircular canals that form loops through the temporal bone. Together, the utricle, saccule, and semicircular canals are thought to play a role in the symptoms associated with vestibular migraine – particularly vertigo and dizziness – and as such we will look closely at the anatomy of each of these structures.

Saccule

The saccule is a bulged-out portion of the labyrinth responsible for detecting vertical motion of the head. For example, jumping up and down or riding in an elevator are activities that activate the motion sensors within the saccule. The saccule lies near the bottom of the vestibule structure, close to the entrance of the cochlea.

Within the saccule is a structure called the *macula sacculi*, a vertically-oriented organ which houses a two- to three-millimeter area comprised of sensory hair cells responsible for detecting head motion. The ends of these hair cells extend horizontally into the middle of the vestibule and are covered by a gelatinous layer, over which is a fibrous structure called the otolithic membrane. This otolithic membrane is embedded with thousands of crystals known by a variety of names including *statoconia, otoconia,* and the aforementioned *otolith*. For the purpose of this book we will use the term *otolith* to describe the crystals of the ear.

Because it is embedded with calcium-based otoliths, the otolithic membrane is heavier than the structures around it. Therefore, when the body moves somewhat quickly in a vertical plane such as occurs when jumping, gravity pulls the otoliths downward the same way as a branch might bend when you swing it upward. The weight of the embedded otoliths causes the hair cells in the otolithic membrane to bend in response to linear motion, thereby sending a signal to the brain that is interpreted as vertical movement of the head.

Utricle

The utricle has an almost identical makeup as the saccule but has a slightly different orientation and function. The utricle is larger than the saccule and serves to detect when the head moves in the horizontal plane, such as might occur with forward, backward, or side-to-side motion of the head. Motions which activate the utricle include the sensation experienced when taking off in an airplane, or when riding in a car as it turns a corner. Like the saccule, the utricle contains a macula called the *macula utriculi*. In contrast to the saccule's vertically-oriented macula, the macula utriculi is positioned horizontally with hair cells that are oriented vertically. The mechanism by which the macula utriculi detects motion operates similarly to that of the macula sacculi in that the hair cells are covered with a gelatinous layer which is in turn overlaid with a membrane embedded with otoliths.

When forward, backward, or side-to-side head motion occurs, the inertia created from the force of the motion upon the embedded otoliths creates a sort of 'shearing' motion between the gelatinous layer and the otolithic membrane. This motion is then detected by the utricle's hair cells which send a signal to the brain that gets interpreted as the respective directional motion of the head.

Otoliths

Because of the otolith's likely role in vertigo associated with vestibular migraine and positional vertigo, it is relevant to provide a specific overview of what these small crystalline structures are. Otoliths are microscopic (approximately 0.0004 inches long), calcium carbonate structures of the inner ear. This chemical makeup of otoliths – calcium carbonate – is effectively the same structure as limestone, and serves to provide weight to the crystals.

As we have discussed, these otoliths are embedded within the otolithic membrane. When the head is not moving the otolithic membrane is stationary and the brain does not receive any significant signal from the hair cells located in the layer underneath the otolithic membrane. When the head moves, however, that motion causes the otolithic membrane to lag slightly behind due to the accumulated weight of the otoliths. Think of this in terms of how when you press hard on the accelerator in your car, your motion of being pressed back into the driver's seat is just slightly delayed. The weight of the otoliths cause a similarly slight delay in saccule and utricle motion within the vestibule. The brain then senses this slight lag and interprets the resulting signal in order to determine directional head movement and force.

Otoliths have a small amount of protein within their structure, and this protein's function is to help the otolith anchor adequately to the otolithic membrane[3]. However, certain conditions can cause the otolith to become dislodged from the otolithic membrane. For example, head trauma can physically displace otoliths from the membrane. And, it has been shown that otoliths degenerate over time, and this degeneration tends to increase with age[4]. This degeneration decreases the anchoring of the otolith to the otolithic membrane[5]. Consequently, otoliths in the process of degenerating can become dislodged from the otolithic

28

membrane and be released into the endolymphatic space of the utricle or saccule in response to a very mild force[6]. Separately, it has been suggested that a change in the pH of the fluid within the labyrinth system may also contribute to allowing otoliths to detach from the otolithic membrane[7]. When displacement of otoliths occurs, they are allowed to move freely around the labyrinth system of the inner ear and have the potential to cause vertigo and/or dizziness such as occurs in the relatively common condition of BPPV.

Semicircular Canals

In addition to the saccule and utricle, there are three semicircular canals of the inner ear's labyrinth network that make up the remainder of the vestibular system. Like the cochlea, the semicircular canals exist as three 'tunnels' or canals through the temporal bone. Membranes line the bone-encased semicircular canals and serve to contain the endolymph fluid that exists throughout the labyrinth system. Like each maculi of the utricle and saccule, motions of the head cause the endolymph to move within the canals as we will discuss shortly. As the movement of endolymph flows across specialized sensors, signals are sent to the brain which interpret the direction of head movement. Whereas the saccule and utricle detect 'linear' movement such as acceleration or vertical motion, the semicircular canals detect 'angular' movement. An example of angular movement would be that type of motion occurring when turning the head side-to-side as if watching a tennis match. Because this movement does not generate forces that act upon the saccule or utricle, the design of the semicircular canals can detect this angular motion and provide feedback to the brain regarding the type of movement.

There are three independent semicircular canals that serve to provide feedback about head position. These three canals are designated the anterior, posterior, and horizontal canals. Based on their position, the three canals are effectively placed at right angles to each other which in turn allows all head motions to be detected. This design can be imagined by thinking of a corner of a cube – each of the three sides of the cube outlines a different plane of movement and are positioned at right angles to each other.

In terms of structure and function of the canals, the anterior canal is positioned higher than the other two canals and is responsible for detecting motions such as occur when nodding one's head. Think back to the utricle for a moment. As we discussed, for motion to be detected by the utricle there needs to be horizontal force capable of causing that 'lag' within the gel layer. Nodding one's head does not generate enough inertia to necessarily cause that lag to occur; however, it does cause a small movement of endolymph within the appropriate semicircular canal. This is why even though both the utricle and sacculi detect motion, we need semicircular canals to detect those small movements that don't necessarily occur in a linear direction. Another example would be rapidly shaking the head to signal 'no'. This small motion wouldn't likely trigger the utricle adequately, but can still be detected by the horizontal canal. The third canal – the posterior – sits lower than the other two canals and serves to detect motion such as might occur if you touch one of your ears to its same-side shoulder.

So how does movement of fluid within the semicircular canals actually result in the brain being able to detect the motion? It's quite a fascinating process (at least in my mind!), actually. Angular motion is detected due to endolymph passing over a specialized organ within each canal called the *cupula*. Movement of the head in an angular motion (i.e. shaking the head 'no', nodding the head, etc.) causes movement of endolymph, which in turn flows across hair cells that move in response to the pressure of the moving fluid. These hair cells are located within the canal itself, at each end of the semicircular canal in an area called the *ampulla* (see Figure 1.3). The ampulla is a bulged-out area of the semicircular canal near the utricle. Hair cells within the ampulla contain the cupula, a gelatinous layer over the hair cells that extends across the width of the ampulla.

As we discussed, when a person moves his or her head the endolymph moves within the semicircular canal in response to the head movement. As the fluid moves, it flows around the cupula (Figure 1.4). As the motion of the endolymph pushes against the cupula, the cupula bends. This causes hair cells immediately under the cupula to also bend, the same way we described that tree branch bending if its leafy end were placed into flowing water. This bending of the hair cells sends a signal to the brain which is interpreted as motion appropriate to the direction of head movement.

These events occurring within the semicircular canals are important to understand, as they are largely thought to play a role in vertigo and dizziness. As far back as the 1960s, researchers believed that conditions such as BPPV – which triggers bouts of vertigo, nystagmus (rapid eye motion), and unsteadiness – resulted from otoliths acting upon the cupula within the semicircular canal[8]. It was suspected even back then that BPPV itself resulted from otoliths actually adhering

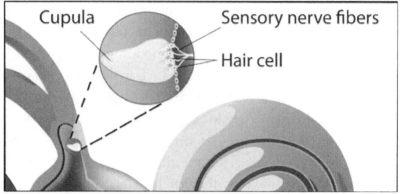

Figure 1.4.   The cupula resides within the ampulla of each semicircular canal. Movement of endolymph causes the cupula to bend, thereby activating the underlying hair cells.

to or interfering with the normal motion of the cupula, in turn causing the cupula to become heavier (due to the added weight of the otoliths) or at least making it perform differently, thereby increasing its sensitivity to motion of the fluid within the semicircular canal[9].

Vertigo and the vestibular system

If you're wondering why we went into such detail regarding the vestibular system, the answer is two-fold. One reason is that I want you to have an understanding of the complexity of the vestibular system and the semicircular canals that we rely on to maintain balance and interpret motion. As we have shown, this system is highly complex. Even small disruptions to the system can have a significant impact on several aspects of our life. This in turn leads to the second reason I wanted to outline the vestibular system in depth – vertigo.

Vertigo is the sensation of movement when in fact no movement is occurring. It is important to understand that vertigo is a symptom, not an actual medical condition; therefore, expecting a cure for vertigo is effectively the same as expecting a cure for pain. What is likely meant is expecting a cure for what is *causing* the pain. The inner ear is thought to play a significant role in vertigo, and has been identified as the source of certain inner-ear conditions that can trigger vertigo, such as BPPV. But other conditions are not as clear cut, and are thought to involve a complex interaction between the brain (i.e. 'central' vertigo) and the inner ear (i.e. 'peripheral' vertigo).

For patients, it is important to understand that vertigo has several possible sources, and no one event or structure has been established as the cause for vertigo. However, researchers have largely narrowed peripheral vertigo down to the semicircular canals, saccule, or utricle, while central vertigo is typically associated with either the brainstem or the vestibulocochlear nerve[10]. Normally, the inner ear structures send signals to the brain in a coordinated pattern from the left and right ear. However, an imbalance of these vestibular inputs leads to uncoordinated information being transmitted to the brain, in turn triggering vestibular nystagmus or vertigo to occur. The imbalanced signal can occur due to disruption anywhere along the pathway that exists from the vestibular-based sensors all the way to the brain.

As stated earlier, there is no specific structure or area that triggers vertigo across all patients. For example, a benign tumor along the vestibulocochlear nerve, known as a vestibular schwanomma or "acoustic neuroma", can be a source of vertigo. Separately, patients experiencing migraine also report vertigo, much like those more commonly recognized patients with disorders specific to the vestibule of the inner ear. The lack of a specific structure being identified as responsible for vertigo development has led some researchers to also include cervical vertigo, or that vertigo arising from degrading intervertebral discs, as an additional source of vertigo[11]. Though cervical-based issues may not fit the traditional idea of vertigo causes, remember that vertigo is a symptom; therefore, it does not have a single cause in the same way that pain can come in many forms (e.g. burning, stinging, sharp, etc.) and locations.

Given the fact that vertigo often affects our balance, there is good reason to suspect that vertigo is largely due to an issue within the inner ear. There is actually a specific set of guidelines that can be applied toward identifying the cause of vertigo. These guidelines outline the use of signs such as the direction of eye movement or the length of time the vertigo lasts in order to establish whether it is central or peripheral in nature[12]. But the interpretation of vertigo is beyond the scope of this book; rather, the analysis of one's vertigo should occur in consultation with a trained medical professional.

One problem that these professionals have in establishing vertigo as a symptom is that patients often lump it in with dizziness. Both vertigo and dizziness are indeed similar in their effects given that each can make the patient

34

feel unsteady. One recommended way to separate the two conditions is to establish whether the patient feels lightheaded or whether they feel as though the world is 'spinning'. Generally, a spinning sensation is more characteristic of vertigo, while lightheadedness is typically associated with dizziness[13]. Further investigation into the type of dizziness often reveals that the patient seems to be either spinning within their environment (internal vertigo) or having their environment spin around them instead (external vertigo). This sensation is largely due to the link between the inner ear and the eyes. In fact, this link plays a vital role in our daily function even though we may not recognize it (unless there is a problem!). To outline this role, we need to discuss the vestibulo-ocular reflex (VOR) and how it coordinates the interaction between the ear and eye.

The vestibulo-ocular reflex (VOR)

The eyes are intimately tied in with the inner ear, and this interaction plays an important role in your ability to maintain balance. To see how important your vision is for aiding in your balance, walk quickly from a bright room into a very dark one. You'll probably find that you are timid and a little bit unsteady, which will likely improve once your eyes adjust to the darkness. Because the vestibular system of the inner ear is also tied into the movement of the eyes, it's relevant to include a discussion of the physiology of this link, or the 'vestibulo-ocular reflex', in this chapter given your recent introduction to the vestibular system. We won't go deep into the details of how the VOR works, but we will provide a general overview of the reflex as it relates to a few expected symptoms of vestibular migraine.

If you've had vertigo in conjunction with vestibular migraine you've no doubt had the uneasy experience of watching objects in your field of view float around or even flash back and forth. This is one of the unfortunate complications of having a vestibular disorder. Many individuals with vestibular disorders notice strange and often frustrating things occurring with their eyes or their vision even though they have a disorder that largely affects their inner ear. Such examples include a rapid and uncontrolled movement of the eyes (i.e. nystagmus) during an attack, or the classic vertigo complaint of the room appearing to be spinning around.

Believe it or not, neither your vision nor your balance systems are independent in how they function; rather, they are each tied into each other in a way that until being affected by vestibular migraine or some other inner-ear disorder, you may not have even recognized. Their interconnection is what allows you to maintain a smooth, non-jumpy field of vision while running or riding on a bumpy road. This happens because the vestibular system actually has some control over the muscle of the eyes via the VOR that allows your eyes to remain fixed on an object even though your head position may be moving. This reflex has the task of trying to ensure that an image or object remains stable on an individual's retina in order to allow for proper processing by the brain[14]. Without the VOR, every time your head moves, you would consciously need to readjust your eye position back to the object you are looking at. With the VOR, however, your vestibular system is able to detect the speed of your head motion and automatically control the muscles in your eye so that your gaze easily remains fixed on the object. This reflex also works well when driving, as every time you hit a bump or turn a corner your eyes are easily controlled rather than jumping all around – which would certainly be a problem when operating a vehicle!

When the VOR is working correctly you don't even know that it's there. But when there is a disruption to the system, such as occurs in response to a vestibular-related disease, the VOR becomes impaired and can lead to uncontrolled movements such as the aforementioned nystagmus. Consequently, an affected patient is not able to coordinate their eye movements with the movements of their head. This can lead to jumpy or blurry vision, likely occurring most often when the head is moving or the patient's body is in motion. Another condition that can result is *oscillopia* in which objects appear to 'bounce' around even though they are in fact stationary, as the muscles of the eye cannot stay adequately fixed on the object.

Additional problems occur when a person with a faulty VOR tries to follow movement or try to read text on paper or a computer screen. With the VOR not allowing for smooth eye movement such as that required to follow a thrown ball or read printed text, it can be difficult for the patient to make the smooth eye motions needed to properly intake visual information (i.e. interpret the written words or follow the ball). Without a well-established link between our eyes and our ears, life would be much more difficult. But unfortunately, because of this link between our eyes and ears we must pay the price of often having visual disturbances such as vertigo or nystagmus when our vestibular system is malfunctioning.

Summary

Because vertigo is intricately tied into the structures of the inner ear, this chapter's orientation to the involved anatomy was intended to help outline those structures that play a major role in the events involved in vertigo and dizziness. Knowing how the physiology of the inner ear works can in turn help explain many of the effects (unsteadiness, nystagmus, etc.) associated with vertigo-type events like vestibular migraine. In the next chapter, we'll investigate the second major component of vestibular migraine – migraine itself – in order to better understand the underlying causes of migraine along with who is affected. This will then set us up to take an in-depth look at the condition of vestibular migraine, as we can draw from both our overview of vestibular anatomy as well as suspected migraine causes in order to understand the complexity of what is occurring during a vestibular migraine attack.

Chapter 2: Migraine

TRADITIONALLY, MOST PEOPLE THINK of a migraine as simply a severe headache. From one aspect they are correct in that headache is a component of migraine, which is a type of 'primary headache disorder' that also includes tension-type and cluster headaches within the classification. However, the definition and classification of migraine has changed over the years and is now a much more complex event than just a headache. Now, migraines can be classified based on location in addition to duration. In this chapter we'll take a very broad and basic look at migraine itself in order to form an understanding of what migraine is as well as the typical symptoms that a migraine sufferer can experience. This will help set up the next chapter that looks specifically at vestibular migraine, an even more complex disorder that often involves migraine in conjunction with some aspect of the vestibular system such as vertigo or unsteadiness. As we will see, migraine itself can be an extremely debilitating condition, made worse by the significant impact of the vestibular system. By first outlining these two individual components of vestibular migraine, it should help provide a foundation that allows us to better understand the next chapter of this book that discusses the vestibular migraine itself.

What is Migraine

At its most basic level, migraine is a severe headache. The American Migraine Foundation outlines a person as having migraine if they've experienced *5 or more attacks of unprovoked headache lasting 4-72 hours, severe enough to markedly restrict or even prohibit routine daily activity and accompanied by nausea or light/sound sensitivity*[15]. As classified, migraine is as much about impact on daily life as it is about severity of the pain. There is no *aura* – or 'warning' – of an impending headache required for a migraine to exist, and the headache itself does not have to be disabling. In fact, a headache is not required to occur each time an aura occurs[15].

Migraine has been outlined as a recurrent headache disorder that affects from approximately 10 - 15% of the population between the ages of 22 and 55[16, 17]. However, the actual prevalence of migraine is expected to be higher as it has been stated that up to 50% of individuals with migraine go undiagnosed or are incorrectly treated for sinus issues or other non-migraine types of headache[18]. Females have been shown to be affected by migraine from 1.5 to 5 times more than males[19, 20] and as it can run in families it is considered a genetic disorder[21]. Children can also be impacted by migraine, with prevalence affecting kids at increasing rates from the age of 3 all the way through adolescence[22]. Because of the range of symptoms associated with migraine it is no longer considered 'just a headache'; rather, it has been outlined as a *complex neurological disorder that affects multiple cortical, subcortical, and brainstem areas that regulate autonomic, affective, cognitive, and sensory functions*[23]. Because of the complexities involved with migraine, in order to begin to unlock the range of events occurring prior to, during, and after migraine, researchers must take into account how a variety of neural networks interact with brain functions and how these networks can be triggered by issues such as stress, hormonal changes, skipping meals, flashing lights, and others[23].

Cause of Migraine

Despite vast advances in medicine over the past 50 years, the events involved in migraine are still not well understood. It is generally accepted that migraine involves the brain, and migraine itself is often described as a neurovascular disorder of the brain[24]. One of the unique problems with migraine is that the events preceding a migraine attack are thought to also increase the susceptibility to triggers[25, 26]. In other words, the period prior to a migraine serves to allow certain events such as stressful situations to more easily elicit a full migraine attack.

One theory behind the precise cause of migraine suggests that there is a set of specific electrical-based events (i.e. depolarization) followed by a period of suppressed brain activity[27]. This process, known as *cortical spreading depression* (CSD), or 'Leao spreading depression', involves a complex array of biochemical processes involving ions and molecules such as potassium, calcium, sodium, and adenosine triphosphate (ATP)[28]. The intricacies of CSD are quite intricate and as a result will not be outlined in detail in this book. Yet it is also important to understand that CSD as a mechanism for migraine has not been proven and therefore remains hypothetical only[1].

There are several other theories as to the cause of migraine. These include hypersensitive pain receptors[29], increased inflammatory markers brought about by constriction and dilation of arteries within the skull[30], genetic influences[31], and even structural changes within the brain[32]. If you are interested in reading more about the suspected causes and underlying events associated with migraine, there are a wealth of books available which are dedicated specifically to migraine.

Phases of migraine

Traditionally, there are four phases to migraine: premonitory, aura, headache, and postdrome. Some individuals experience these four phases in sequence while others experience significant overlap between the phases[24]. The premonitory, or 'premonition', phase involves a set of symptoms that occur up to 72 hours prior to the actual headache include food cravings, yawning, stiff neck, and/or photophobia (i.e. hypersensitivity to light), among others[24, 33]. The aura phase, experienced by approximately one-fourth to one-third of migraine sufferers[34, 35] involves a period of neurological deficit that can last between five and sixty minutes[24] and may include visual symptoms such as spots floating in one's eye and, to a lesser extent, sensory aura that includes numbness or tingling in the extremities or face[34]. For other individuals, the headache itself has no aura and therefore begins without warning, often ending with sleep[23]. However, the headache can also be triggered by events such as fatigue, euphoria, depression, irritability, or sensitivity to light and/or sound[36].

The third phase of a migraine – the headache phase – involves a period of time from 4-72 hours during which two of the following conditions must be met: located on one side, pulsating, moderate to severe in intensity, and aggravated by physical activity[24]. The most common type of migraine is known as *migraine without aura* which includes symptoms of headache, nausea, vomiting, and sensitivity to both light and sound[37]. During an attack, the patient can be affected for anywhere from 4 to 72 hours and may require bedrest[34]. The actual migraine itself is limited to one side of the head (i.e. unilateral), pulsating in nature, and typically increases in severity during physical activity[37]. The migraine can also include additional effects that are physical in nature such as nausea, vomiting, congestion, and even diarrhea, as well as psychological and cognitive effects such as irritability, depression, and transient amnesia[38].

The last phase of a migraine, the postdrome, involves the after-effects of the migraine which can include tiredness, difficulty concentrating, and neck stiffness[24]. Interestingly, migraine sufferers often attribute many of these postdrome symptoms to the medication used to treat the migraine rather than as a component of the migraine itself [24].

43

Financial Impact of Migraine

Migraine is quite costly, with the most recent data indicating that the annual cost for migraine per person in the United States is $2,649[39] and the total cost on the United States in 1999 dollars at $13.3 billion[40]. Migraine is listed as the sixth most disabling condition worldwide, and the most disabling neurological disorder[33]. Even more worrisome is that its position on these disorder rankings is rising, which suggests that migraine is slowly affecting more of the population over time[41, 42].

Risk factors for Migraine

While the first symptom of migraine is often the migraine itself, certain risk factors have been identified that can predispose an individual to having migraine attacks. For example, an overuse of acute migraine medication, described as *intake of analgesics more than 15 days a month or triptans more than 10 days per month* has been shown to trigger an increase in headache frequency[43, 44]. Ironically, stopping the overuse of headache medication has also been shown to significantly ease the individual's headache[45]. This evidence suggests that there is an 'upper limit' at which medication should be taken for migraine, as taking medication for extended periods of time (i.e. 'overuse') can actually increase one's risk for developing migraine.

Outside of a medication aspect, obese individuals are more likely to suffer from migraines[46] as well as suffer more migraines per month[47]. Additionally, depression – as well as the severity of the depression – also increases the risk for migraine[48]. Stressful life events such as divorce can also serve to increase one's risk for suffering from migraine[43].

Migraine Treatment

Treatment of migraine largely focuses on two goals – stopping current attacks and preventing future attacks. One of the first preventative tactics is to avoid those risk factors that increase your chances for developing chronic migraine. While prevention is best, it is not always effective as it can be difficult for an individual to avoid all risk factors. Furthermore, acute migraines can still occur even with preventative treatments.

Drug treatment for migraine often involves beta-blockers, topiramate, or valproate, each of which has been shown to be effective for treating migraine[49]. Acute migraine attacks have resulted in the development of the drug triptan which can be effective for ending or at least diminishing a migraine that is occurring. Drugs that target specific antibodies, including those of the trigeminal nerve that is thought to be involved in migraine, are currently under development and appear to show some promise for improving migraine treatment[50], as an injection of this drug type can prevent or at least reduce migraine attacks over the following three months[23]. However, as mentioned earlier, the known occurrence of medication overuse as a risk factor for migraine is important given the fact that medication is often successfully used to treat and prevent migraine[43]. To address this issue of overuse, one panel of experts recommended preventative treatment in combination with short-term use of medication[51].

Besides pharmaceutical intervention, therapies which target those brain modifications (e.g. structural and electrophysiological changes) shown to occur in migraine patients are also under development. One treatment known as transcranial magnetic stimulation is thought to alter hyper-excitability of the cortical brain area[52]. Separately, cognitive behavioral therapy is under investigation to see if thought processes and attitudes can play a role in altering the severity or duration of migraine[53].

Conclusion

Migraine is an intermittent headache disorder that affects approximately 15% of the population, most often between 22 and 55 years of age[16]. It is thought to be neurogenic in nature and can present itself in varying degrees of severity for sufferers. Migraine can be a significant hindrance on daily life for many patients and is even one of the leading causes of suicide[54]. Currently, diagnosis is dependent upon the patient's symptoms and family history, and evidence indicates that migraine has a favorable but not universal response to treatments such as medication.

Chapter 3: Vestibular Migraine

TO UNDERSTAND WHAT A VESTIBULAR migraine is, we first had to outline the two conditions that make up its name. Therefore, in the previous chapters we briefly discussed much of the vestibular system of the inner ear as well as what a migraine is. This in turn provides us at least a basic understanding of the structures that play a significant role in the development of vertigo and dizziness along with the general evidence for what is thought to cause a migraine. Understanding what a migraine is becomes central to understanding the condition known as vestibular migraine. In this chapter, we'll take a look at the research surrounding vestibular migraine in order to help you better understand the condition, who it affects, and what is suspected to be occurring as a result of vestibular migraine. Despite our relatively recent classification of vestibular migraine, we have come far in understanding many of the events involved. In reading this chapter, you can expect to gain a better understanding of the events involved in your own vestibular migraine, and by being aware of the most recent research you can hopefully have a constructive conversation with your physician in order to get on or continue your path to successful treatment.

Defining Vestibular Migraine

As we have outlined, vertigo and migraine can exist as separate medical conditions. They can also, however, occur at the same time and in turn require a unique medical designation. Historically, several different names have been used to outline the simultaneous occurrence of vertigo and migraine, including migrainous vertigo, migraine-associated vertigo, migraine-associated dizziness, migraine-related vestibulopathy, benign recurrent vertigo, and basilar migraine[55]. The lack of consistency in describing the same general medical condition we now know as vestibular migraine highlights the fact that for a long time there was no clear diagnostic criteria for vestibular migraine, and that the complexity of the disorder could make for a difficult diagnosis[1]. Over time it has been suggested that the term 'vestibular migraine' best avoids conflict or confusion with other, non-vestibular types of dizziness that are also associated with migraine[56]. Furthermore, 'vestibular migraine' is the term utilized by the Bárány Society as well as the International Headache Society, and their joint classification of the disease also specifically uses the term 'vestibular migraine'.

History of Vestibular Migraine

Even though it is generally accepted that vestibular migraine is itself a relatively new medical condition, the events involved in vestibular migraine are well documented. Historically speaking, Aretaeus of Cappadocia has been credited with first outlining vestibular symptoms in conjunction with a migraine back in 131 AD[57]. In more modern times, physician Edward Lieving back in 1873 outlined a link between migraine and vertigo[58]. Then in the early 1960s, migraine was for the first time described as occurring in conjunction with symptoms arising from the brainstem in a condition outlined as *basilar artery migraine*[57].

The first reported description of what we now know as vestibular migraine is credited to researchers Kayan and Hood who back in 1984 described a syndrome that combined headache, vertigo, and visual events[59]. This term was later renamed as *migraine with brainstem aura*[37]. The actual term 'vestibular migraine' was first used by Boenheim back in 1999[60], and this description has remained as the term of choice for the past two decades.

Prevalence of Vestibular Migraine

Prevalence is a term used to describe how widespread an illness is, and is usually reported as either a percent of the population with a condition or a ratio of having a disease versus all people in a population (e.g. 1 in 250 people). Determining the true prevalence of vestibular migraine can be somewhat difficult because of the individual conditions –

vertigo and migraine – that make up vestibular migraine. In other words, a person can have a vestibule-related problem such as dizziness or vertigo but can also have a separate history of migraine. If the two aren't associated, that individual does not have vestibular migraine even though he or she may be exhibiting the main symptoms of the condition. This outlines the difficulty in determining prevalence of vestibular migraine, as the two conditions aren't always linked; therefore it can be challenging to establish whether a patient has true 'vestibular migraine' or if they instead have dizziness separate from a migraine. Therefore, it is always important that evaluation for vestibular migraine is conducted by a trained medical professional so that these other conditions do not influence a patient's ultimate diagnosis.

Specific to prevalence of vestibular migraine in patients, one nearly twenty year-old study found that among 200 patients who entered a 'dizziness clinic', 7% had what was considered to be a vestibular migraine. Similarly, a migraine-specific clinic found that 9% of patients ended up being classified as having vestibular migraine[61]. This evidence suggests that of individuals who seek treatment for a migraine, nearly 1 in 10 actually have a vestibular migraine. However, any prevalence value relating to vestibular migraine must be viewed with caution, as it has been reported that only about 2 out of 3 patients with dizziness disorders visit their physician[62]. But as we will discuss, of those that do seek medical attention for dizziness, vestibular migraine is rarely suspected initially.

Lifetime prevalence is another way to look at how much a disease or condition affects a population. As a descriptor, lifetime prevalence differs a little bit from overall prevalence of a disease in that it describes the proportion of a population that has experienced a particular disorder at some point in their life. For example, the lifetime prevalence of anxiety disorders has been reported to be 35%[63], meaning that 35% of whatever population was studied (e.g. 'adults in the United States') has had an anxiety disorder at some point in their life. Migraines have a lifetime prevalence of 14%[64], and vertigo resulting from a vestibular condition has a lifetime prevalence of 7%[65]. Because the two conditions must exist together in order to have a diagnosis of vestibular migraine, it would be expected that the lifetime prevalence of having both conditions would theoretically be around 1.1%[66], or that approximately 1 in 100 people would be expected to have vestibular migraine during their life. One study that used an actual patient population found that the lifetime prevalence of vestibular migraine was actually around 3.2%, a value almost three times higher than that predicted from separate vertigo and migraine calculations[67]!

Epidemiology of Vestibular Migraine

Epidemiology looks at causes and trends in patients and populations in an attempt to find potential causes of a disease. With vestibular migraine, current epidemiological reports are probably not representative of the true characteristics of the disease given that vestibular migraine has been shown to be under-diagnosed. Evidence for this stems from the fact that in one study, 20.2% of patients were ultimately diagnosed with vestibular migraine, but less than

2% of doctors who had referred those patients actually suspected vestibular migraine[68]. This finding highlights the importance of getting a correct diagnosis of vestibular migraine from the proper medical professional in order to apply adequate treatment. Not surprisingly, this low rate of diagnosis was suspected to be due to what we have already discussed – the fact that vestibular migraine symptoms often mimic other vertigo-inducing conditions[69].

While some vertigo-associated conditions such as Ménière's disease tend to increase in frequency later in life, vestibular migraine can occur at effectively any age[70 71]. The age of onset for vestibular migraine can range from 7 to 74 years and does include children as we will discuss in a later chapter[72]. The average age, though, at which vestibular migraine symptoms begin for adults has been reported as 37.7 years for women and 42.4 years for men[61].

Women have been shown to experience vestibular migraine at a much higher rate than men, at a 1.5 to 5-times higher occurrence[61, 70]. This higher vestibular migraine rate in females mimics the higher female rate shown to occur for traditional migraine as well[70]. Is has been suggested that this higher rate in women is thought to be due in part to a genetic factor of vestibular migraine, specifically some yet-unknown factor that is suppressed at a greater rate in men[73]. Evidence also indicates that women often see a change from migraine headaches to migraine-based vertigo attacks around the time of menopause[74].

Cause of Vestibular Migraine

Despite an increased focus on vestibular migraine over the past two decades, the true underlying factors involved in the development of vestibular migraine remain to be determined and continue to be a subject of debate[69]. Many times, the cause of vestibular migraine is incorrectly attributed to migraine itself; however, classifying the symptoms as being associated with migraine does not account for the vestibular aspects such as dizziness and vertigo[1]. As we outlined previously, it's certainly possible that there are two separate events going on – vertigo and migraine – but it also must be taken into account that the vertigo is directly attributable to the migraine[65], indicating that vestibular migraine is the true culprit.

It is believed that there is a significant neural and/or neurovascular cause behind many of the symptoms of vestibular migraine[24]. This is a bit of a modification from older theories that tied symptoms into a strictly vascular cause[24]. For example, it was long thought that vestibular migraine-type symptoms were the result of brain stem ischemia (i.e. restriction of blood flow). This belief resulted in terminology such as *vascular headache* and *basilar artery migraine* being used to describe headaches that involved dizziness[57, 75]. Now, however, the prevailing thought is that there is a neural *and* likely vascular cause for vestibular migraine[24].

Because a vestibular migraine typically involves vertigo as well as headache, it is believed that there is both peripheral (i.e. inner ear) and central-type (i.e. brain) vestibular involvement that influences the symptoms of vestibular migraine[76]. This theory is due in part to the fact that several neurochemical transmitters are required for physiological processes that involve both migraine development and vestibular function[77]. As such, any disruption or improper signaling from these neurotransmitters could result in simultaneous symptoms being exhibited from both the vestibular system and the brain, as has been shown to occur with vestibular migraine. For example, researchers have found that there is a link between nocioceptors (i.e. painful or harmful stimuli receptors) of the nervous system and the vestibular system[78]. This link could help explain evidence indicating that patients with vestibular migraine exhibit increased signal transmission between their nocioceptors and vestibular systems compared to that of healthy people[1]. And because the migraine component of vestibular migraine often occurs with pain[79], the involvement of nocioceptors is certainly possible.

Additional evidence for a neural cause behind vestibular migraine has been shown using nerve stimulation. The trigeminal nerve – one of several cranial nerves located at the base of the brain – is responsible for both vestibular-based neural signaling and for playing a role in regulating blood flow to the inner ear[80]. It has been shown that when applying intense electrical stimulation to the area of facial skin innervated by the trigeminal nerve, nystagmus was triggered in vestibular migraine patients but not in healthy individuals[81]. Because nystagmus is often attributed to vestibular involvement, and because vestibular migraine patients often exhibit nystagmus[82], this finding lends evidence that the trigeminal nerve may at least have some role in vestibular migraine symptoms.

Further evidence for a neural involvement in vestibular migraine stems from the fact that patients often have a hyperactive vestibular system that may be more susceptible to movement-type inputs such as head tilting[83, 84]. A reason for this hypersensitive response is not yet known. Another theory suggests that a cause for vestibular migraine is tied into a neurochemical response that may also involve blood flow similar to what happens with migraine[85]. Certain chemical triggers of migraine such as nitroglycerin can cause an increased sensitivity to the blood vessels of the outermost membrane (i.e. dural) of the brain. Because this ties into blood flow to the brain, it is suspected that this link between certain chemical agents and blood supply in the brain might explain why activities that are normally tolerable – such as exercise or coughing – can suddenly increase the presence of headache in migraine, and might partially explain why migraine pain is often described as 'throbbing'[24]. But again, this vascular-based theory does not account for the vertigo often associated with vestibular migraine.

There are many other suspected causes – revealed through detailed research beyond the scope of this book – that are suspected to play a role in vestibular migraine. These suspected causes can be both internal to the body such as genetic involvement or outside of the body like those that can occur due to certain triggers or the environment[78]. All vestibular migraine causes though, are largely theoretical and therefore require significant additional research to be carried out in order to establish a more definitive cause. And, improved technology will go a long way towards helping to determine what is happening with vestibular migraine. For example, in recent years, improvements in technology have allowed imaging to become more useful in unlocking the cause of vestibular migraine. Some researchers have in turn been able to focus on a certain area of the brain called the thalamus, as magnetic resonance imaging (MRI) indicate an increase in thalamus activity among vestibular migraine sufferers[86]. Furthermore, imaging has allowed for the detection of small structural changes in patients with vestibular migraine. Researchers have found evidence of an increase in the brain's gray matter among vestibular migraine patients[87], suggesting that vestibular migraine may actually trigger a physical alteration of tissue in the brain.

Despite the fact that there has yet to be a clear cut mechanism behind vestibular migraine, it is important for patients to understand that this doesn't mean that a cause is not lurking just out of our reach. Remember that in the realm of headache or dizziness-type conditions, vestibular migraine is one of the more recently recognized medical conditions, and therefore it has been subjected to a shorter investigational timeframe compared to other vestibular disorders. It's important to remember that with each small discovery, though, another piece of the puzzle gets added to the overall picture of curing vestibular migraine. So even though a particular research study may not reveal a new potential cause for vestibular migraine, it may reveal a unique characteristic specific to vestibular migraine patients that we did not know previously. Researchers could then focus in on this new finding and conduct more studies that could potentially reveal a cause – or even a cure – for vestibular migraine. Then once that cause is found, treatments can be developed to help cure or at least reduce the severity of vestibular migraine. Patients must also remember that the lack of a specific identified cause is not uncommon in vestibular ailments, as conditions such as Ménière's disease, suspected to be tied to a series of events in the inner ear, also do not have an identified cause as to why they typically trigger violent vertigo attacks along with often continuous unsteadiness and dizziness.

Symptoms of Vestibular Migraine

Outlining those symptoms specifically associated with vestibular migraine can be a bit complicated because there are no clear set of symptoms that are consistent among all patients. Symptoms such as headache, vertigo, or dizziness are quite common among almost all people at some point. Consequently, it can be difficult for medical professionals to determine whether an individual has vestibular migraine or whether they simply have a headache, an ear infection, or some other common condition that triggers similar symptoms. Therefore, we'll look at some of the more common symptoms associated with vestibular migraine as well as a few of the less-common ones that patients report.

When we look at symptoms, it is important to outline that there are effectively two phases to having vestibular migraine – the 'attack' phase and the 'non-attack' phase. Attacks are acute events during which the majority of symptoms arise including vertigo, migraine, nystagmus, and others. The non-attack phase is that period during which symptoms are largely suppressed and the attack itself is not occurring, yet the patient may still feel unsteady or dizzy to the point that there is some degree of impact on daily activities.

This dual-phase occurrence with vestibular migraine is similar to other conditions of the inner ear such as Ménière's or BPPV which also involves relatively calm phases intermixed with violent vertigo attacks. Specific to vestibular migraine patients, there has been shown to be quite a bit of variability in how long the attacks last. For example, half of vestibular migraine sufferers report an attack duration of one to two days[67], even though attacks can last longer for some patients[88]. Around 40% of vestibular migraine patients report that their attacks last less than a day, while 12% indicate that their attacks last less than one hour. These attacks, which can take a week or more to recover from, may occur days to years apart, oftentimes with no apparent predictability or pattern[66].

When outlining the symptoms of vestibular migraine, one thing to note is that the majority of vestibular migraine patients do not initially experience symptoms associated with true vestibular migraine; rather, most (~75%) patients go through a period of time where they are initially dealing only with the effects of migraine. Approximately half of vestibular migraine patients claim that more than five years passes between their initial migraine symptoms and the start of their vestibular migraine, while up to 25% of patients go more than ten years before their vestibular migraine symptoms begin after their initial migraine event[89]. Furthermore, some patients report developing vestibular migraine only after their migraines have actually began to decrease over time, which has led researchers and medical professionals to attribute vestibular migraine more to vertigo than to headache itself[88].

Headache

The most common migraine-associated symptom during a vestibular migraine attack is headache[69]. Significant pain can occur with these headaches, as one survey revealed that during an attack, 47.5% of patients experienced dizziness or vertigo, with the average degree of headache pain reaching a level of "7" out of "10" (0 = no pain, 10 = worst pain imaginable)[79].

Having headache as the most common migraine-associated symptom during a migraine attack is not to say that all attacks bring on headache, though. Patients report that approximately 30% of their vestibular migraine attacks do not occur with headache[1]. However, about 25% of vestibular migraine patients state that headache is indeed always present during an attack, while a small portion of patients claim that a headache is actually absent during their attack[90]. Interestingly, patients have also reported that when vertigo is present during an attack their headache is less severe than when the headache occurs without vertigo[91]. Such variation even in the most common of symptoms serves to highlight the difficulty medical professionals can often have in diagnosing vestibular migraine.

Vertigo

Half of all patients who experience the traditional form of migraine report at least occasional dizziness or vertigo[92]. This can complicate the diagnosis of vestibular migraine, as even those who suffer from migraine alone also report occasional vestibular-related problems. In older patients, for example, migraine attacks can be replaced by episodes of vertigo, dizziness, or a temporary feeling of disequilibrium[93]. The reports of vertigo or dizziness are, however, similar to what vestibular migraine sufferers are more commonly subjected to on a daily basis, along with repeated and intense attacks of vertigo that the patient feels are both unpredictable and uncontrollable[94]. In fact, vestibular migraine is considered to be the second-most common cause for vertigo in all patients after benign positional vertigo[66] and is the most common cause for recurrent episodes of spontaneous (i.e. sudden or unexpected) vertigo[95].

Even though vestibular migraine is well-associated with vertigo, the type of vertigo that it can cause also varies between patients. Up to 70% of patients report experiencing positional vertigo at some point while dealing with vestibular migraine, even though the vertigo might not occur during every attack[88]. Two-thirds of vestibular migraine patients report a spontaneous rotary vertigo that can arise at anytime, while 24% of patients indicate that they suffer from positional vertigo that occurs in response to specific body and head positions such as lying down[67]. Some patients even experience spontaneous vertigo that turns into positional vertigo within the same attack[96]. Along these lines, one study reported that 44% of vestibular migraine patients claimed to experience internal-type vertigo, that type in which the patient seems to be spinning within their environment, while just over half report that their vertigo seems to cause their environment to spin around them instead (i.e. 'external' vertigo). The remaining patients indicated a mixed degree of both internal and external vertigo[97]. Similarly, vestibular migraine patients also report experiencing a higher frequency of "visual vertigo", or vertigo triggered by moving images such as those that can occur while driving[98].

Despite all this talk of vertigo, it should be noted that not all vestibular migraine attacks involve vertigo. One study reported that anywhere from one-fourth to one-third of attacks do not involve a vertigo-based event[70]. Despite this inconsistency of vertigo during attacks, all patients with vestibular migraine do report experiencing vertigo at some point[66]. This common complain of vertigo helps separate vestibular migraine from migraine itself, as just 50% of patients who experience migraine report some degree of dizziness or vertigo[92]. Still, the link between migraine itself and vertigo is clear, as migraine patients themselves experience vertigo two to three times more often than healthy patients who do not have headaches[99]. Furthermore, it has been shown that patients diagnosed with migraine were also more likely to have vertigo – as well as vertigo with an accompanying headache – compared to patients without migraine[100].

Other symptoms

Along with vertigo, several known symptoms of vestibular migraine exist, but it is important to point out that not all of the symptoms we discuss will occur with each attack. In terms of these other symptoms, patients can report a range of sensations that are probably more consistent with a description of what they're feeling rather than a specific symptom. Examples of some of these additional sensations that vestibular migraine sufferers commonly report include nausea, vomiting, and a desire to lay flat on the ground[55] as well as a 'swimming' sensation, heavy headedness, or a rocking sensation[101]. In between attacks, the most common symptom is positional nystagmus, reported in 28% of patients. Similarly, 41% of patients reported that eye movement was disturbed[82].

Motion sickness

Though not a specific symptom of existing vestibular migraine, motion sickness does seem to show an association with patients who suffer from vestibular migraine. Over half (54%) of vestibular migraine patients tend to exhibit a susceptibility to motion sickness[102]. This increased susceptibility to motion sickness is consistent with evidence that vestibular migraine patients often experience balance, vision disturbances, or nausea in response to certain motions of the head[71], similar to the proportion of vestibular migraine patients that suffer from positional vertigo[67].

Related symptoms

Besides the aforementioned conditions of headache, vertigo, and a susceptibility to motion sickness, other conditions reported regularly by vestibular migraine patients include nausea, vomiting, and a desire to lay flat on the ground[55]. A caveat with many of these symptoms, however, is that they do not necessarily exist *only* because of vestibular migraine but instead may be the result of pre-existing conditions[55]. Inner-ear-specific symptoms also exist, including tinnitus in up to 33% of sufferers, 'fullness' in the ear in up to 20% of patients, and hearing loss in about 10% of patients[67]. Additionally, about half of vestibular migraine sufferers report photophobia (i.e. hypersensitivity to light) in addition to phonophobia (hypersensitivity to loud sounds)[67].

The wide range of symptoms associated with vestibular migraine can be somewhat problematic for treatment. Due to the spontaneous arrival and elimination of many of these vestibular migraine symptoms, it can be difficult to prove that any lessening of symptoms was due to medication use or treatment rather than the normal course of arrival and suppression of vestibular migraine symptoms.

Psychological aspects

Beyond the physical manifestations of vestibular migraine, patients also have to deal with an array of psychological aspects. Most likely due to the unpredictable and perceived uncontrollability of vestibular migraines, sufferers often report panic-related thoughts along with higher rates of separation- and social-based anxiety[94]. This relationship between migraine, vestibular disorders, and anxiety is actually prevalent enough that a medical condition termed *migraine-anxiety-related dizziness* (MARD) is now recognized[103]. Furthermore, many of these psychological symptoms exist to a higher degree in vestibular migraine patients than in patients experiencing migraine only, indicating that vertigo contributes significantly to the psychological aspects of these patients.

Triggers of Vestibular Migraine

Triggers of a vestibular migraine represent any activity (e.g. exercise) or event (e.g. certain smells) that can cause or amplify the effects of a vestibular migraine attack. It goes without saying that any patient of a disorder as debilitating as vestibular migraine will likely go to great lengths to prevent an attack from occurring. To prevent an attack, or at least help reduce the potential for one to occur, it is important that the patient identify his or her triggers that can play a role in the occurrence of an attack. With vestibular migraines, several 'common' triggers have been reported, but it is also very likely that there are triggers which are unique to each individual patient.

Some of the most common triggers of vestibular migraine include menstruation, stress, or a change in sleeping habits[104], along with sensory-based triggers such as bright lights, intense smells, or noise[66]. Other individuals have even reported triggers resulting from specific foods such as cheese, red wine, or glutamate. Unfortunately, there does not appear to be a consistent trigger that is experienced by a high number of vestibular migraine sufferers; as such, patients should be hypervigilant about paying attention to activity that occurs prior to an attack in order to help identify their own triggers. Furthermore, to help recognize those triggers unique to each person, it is often recommended that individuals keep a daily activity log in order to help identify a pattern in activities that may lead to the onset of a vestibular migraine attack. Some attacks might not occur immediately after interacting with a specific trigger; instead it may take hours or more for certain triggers such as food consumption to cause an attack. Having an activity/food log can help tremendously in identifying some triggers by allowing patients and professionals to look through recent activity for likely triggers.

Conclusion

There has been a wealth of attention given to vestibular migraine over the past thirty years. Research has recognized that vertigo and migraine are not just separate conditions but in many cases are directly linked. The turn of the century led to the first set of diagnostic criteria for vestibular migraine and opened the door for treatments directed specifically at this debilitating condition. The relative 'newness' of vestibular migraine has left researchers and medical professionals with relatively inconsistent data;

therefore, much work remains to be done in order to determine the true populations affected, the specific symptoms associated with vestibular migraine, and the best treatments to lessen symptoms or prevent an attack from occurring. Favorable treatment options now include pharmaceutical intervention in addition to vestibular rehabilitation, though both are not viewed as cures but rather treatments to help reduce the frequency and severity of attacks. Further research is needed to help outline the specific events that cause a vestibular migraine as well as those structures involved in developing the pain and dizziness that can occur.

Chapter 4: Vestibular Migraine in Children

I F VESTIBULAR MIGRAINE WAS consistent with most other vestibular disorders such as Ménière's or BPPV, it would hold true that adults are the population most likely to suffer the associated effects. Vestibular migraine, however, appears to differ somewhat from these other conditions given that the research indicates that children are also susceptible to the effects of multiple vestibular-migraine-related conditions, and these conditions tend to have similar symptoms and effects as what occurs in adults. In this chapter we'll look at the issue of vestibular migraine specific to how it affects children and also take a look at how it develops over time in this age group.

Diagnostic criteria issues in children

The diagnosis of a disease in one population does not always apply to another. For example, attention deficit/hyperactivity disorder (ADHD) diagnosis can depend upon which standards are applied to certain age groups[105]. Vestibular migraine is no different. Even though we noted in the previous chapter that vestibular migraine can affect children, those children are being diagnosed under guidelines developed for adults[55]. While it could be argued that children will have the same general symptoms as adults and could in fact reach the same conclusion specific to whether they have vestibular migraine or not, the accuracy of the application of these adult-based diagnostic criteria in children has not been tested scientifically[106]. Furthermore, children seeking medical attention for vestibular-related disorders tend to have a shorter medical history than adult patients specific to dizziness and/or vertigo, and they may have difficulty in describing the detail of their symptoms[107]. These factors can serve to complicate a medical professional's ability to form a solid clinical diagnosis specific to vestibular migraine in children.

Benign positional vertigo

Though not limited specifically to children, it has been shown that young individuals are more at risk for a condition called *benign paroxysmal vertigo*, or "BPV" (not to be confused with BPPV). The International Classification of Headache Disorders (ICHD) recognizes benign positional vertigo of childhood as a viable condition[55]. Similar to the characteristics of vestibular migraine, BPV is described as *a disorder characterized by recurrent brief attacks of vertigo, occurring without warning and resolving spontaneously, in otherwise healthy children*[37]. The ICHD has established a list of criteria that must be met for a diagnosis of BPV. Those criteria include:

A. At least 5 attacks fulfilling criteria B and C
B. Vertigo occurring without warning, maximal at onset, and resolving spontaneously after minutes to hours without loss of consciousness
C. At least one of the following associated symptoms or signs:
   a. Nystagmus
   b. Ataxia (lack of muscle coordination)
   c. Vomiting
   d. Pallor (pale color)
   e. Fearfulness
D. Normal neurological examination and audiometry

Our understanding of BPV occurrence in children has evolved over the years. Initially, BPV was known as "benign paroxysmal vertigo of childhood" and fell into the grouping of *childhood periodic syndromes that may be precursors to, or associated with, migraine*[108]. The next version classified the condition as *childhood periodic syndromes that are commonly precursors of migraine*[109]. Now, BPV is grouped under *episodic syndromes that may be associated with migraine*, along with its official renaming as "benign paroxysmal vertigo"[107]. It was initially thought that BPV was linked with attacks that start in children prior to their reaching the age of 4 years and resolving by the age of 6[107], but more recent evidence indicates that these spells can last through adolescence[72] or transform into other types of migraine[107].

Epidemiology

Children in the United States aged 3-17 report a one-year prevalence of 5.3% for dizziness and balance issues[110]. It is known that the average age at which symptoms of vestibular migraine are first reported in children is around 14 years of age[111] compared to an average age of greater than 40 years in adults[61]. Interestingly, these particular age points have been pointed out as possible indication of a hormonal influence with vestibular migraine[111].

Specific to vestibular migraine, it has been found that among young individuals (18 years of age or less) that visited a dizziness clinic, the prevalence of BPV or vestibular migraine was 30%. Interestingly, as the age of the child increased in this study, the prevalence of BPV went down while the prevalence of vestibular migraine actually increased[112]! This same study noted that among all children who reported to a dizziness clinic for medical care, vestibular migraine was more prevalent than BPV.

Much like vestibular migraine in adults, in a young population it has been shown that girls are more likely to be diagnosed with vestibular migraine than males[111], although the ratio (1.3:1) shown in children is somewhat smaller than that seen in adult women and men[67]. Among children who are seen at dizziness clinics, the diagnosis of vestibular migraine in children ranges between 17.6 and 58%[113]. This wide range is thought in part to be due to variances in diagnostic criteria as well as differences in the specialty of the clinics involved in that particular study[113].

Vestibular migraine symptoms in children

Vestibular migraine is one of the most common causes of episodic vertigo in children[114]. One study looked specifically at the symptoms of vestibular migraine patients who were 18 years of age or less[111]. There, it was determined that every young patient who met the criteria for vestibular migraine or *probable* vestibular migraine suffered from spinning vertigo. Three out of four reported a feeling of swaying or rocking. One in four stated that they had lightheadedness while 14% claimed that they suffered from imbalance. And like adult sufferers, reported triggers included stress, lack of sleep, diet, and experiencing menstruation.

Headache with dizziness

There is a bit of variation specific to the incidence of headache with vertigo or dizziness in studies involving children. One study reported that approximately 25% of affected children reported vertigo with a simultaneous headache 'most of the time'. Nearly two in three stated that headache existed 'some of the time', while 11% claimed that they never had a headache with their vertigo[111]. Of those with headache, 40% stated that it was located on one side, 32% reported that it had a pulsating tendency, and 7% stated that they had both events occur with their headaches.

Other studies looking specifically at those young patients who noted simultaneous headache and vestibular-related conditions found higher values. For example, one study reported that just over half (54%) of patients reported vertigo with headache, while 73% reported having headache[107]. This was similar to a related study in which 51% reported both headache and dizziness[115] while yet another study reported a value of 60%[116].

Other symptoms

There are a variety of other symptoms reported in children with vestibular migraine, many of which mimic those symptoms found in adult patients as well. For example, photophobia, phonophobia, nausea and vomiting, and visual-based aura are common[111]. And the actual vestibular migraine attack event in children has been shown to have a similar duration as in adults, with attacks lasting anywhere from a few minutes to multiple days, averaging around 12 hours in duration[111]. And like adults, children with migraine and vestibular migraine are more likely to suffer from motion sickness, as half of kids with vestibular migraine have reported motion sickness[107].

Conclusion

Children are susceptible to the effects of vestibular migraine much like adults, though their shorter medical history and inability to clearly outline their symptoms can impede a proper diagnosis. Such constraints may make it difficult for medical professionals to separate out the more common condition of BPV in children. Still, vestibular migraine is quite common within the young population, and they often suffer the same effects as adults.

Chapter 5: Diagnosis

IN ORDER TO DIAGNOSE ANY CONDITION, there must be a set of established and validated guidelines that outline what conditions a person must have in order to receive that diagnosis. Some diagnoses, such as having the flu, are relatively easy as they simply require the physical presence of a material such as flu antibodies. Conditions such as migraine or vestibular migraine, however, do not have a physical element. Furthermore, the symptoms associated with vestibular migraine often mimic other conditions such as Ménière's or even a concussion. Only in recent years have a clear set of diagnostic criteria been established for vestibular migraine, and even then, these criteria have been subjected to – and will likely continue to go through – recommended updates and modifications. Despite any future modification, a diagnosis of vestibular migraine is essential for ensuring that vestibular migraine is successfully identified, another condition is not missed, and to ensure that proper treatment is delivered.

The Bárány society was founded in 1960 in order to "facilitate contacts between basic scientists and clinicians engaged in vestibular research, and to stimulate otoneurological education and research"[117]. This society, made up of an array of basic scientists, otolaryngologists, and neurologists who are committed to vestibular research, has been a tremendous advocate for furthering research related to vestibular migraine. As we will outline shortly, the efforts of the Bárány society have led to the establishment of a set of diagnostic criteria that should be met in order to make a diagnosis of vestibular migraine[55].

While it might seem somewhat 'easy' to put together the definition for a particular medical disorder, doing so haphazardly can invite a variety of problems that ultimately end up affecting the patient through either misdiagnosis or leaving their illness undiagnosed. For example, if a particular medical condition's definition requires very precise and specific guidelines, then many patients will be unfairly excluded for not meeting the exact definition of the disease. Such a situation could arise if, for example, a vestibular migraine diagnosis *required* vertigo events in conjunction with migraine. As we now know, not all migraine attacks occur with vertigo. Under those conditions, even one attack that occurs without a simultaneous migraine would exclude that person from a proper diagnosis of vestibular migraine. Conversely, if a more broad set of requirements is introduced, people who do not have the condition will be incorrectly diagnosed. Such a situation could result if the diagnosis for vestibular migraine were simply 'vertigo during a migraine'. In such a case, what would the diagnosis be for a patient who had migraine for

74

10 years then happened to develop BPPV? If they experienced positional vertigo when leaning over to pick up something off the floor while they were also having a migraine (i.e. vertigo during a migraine), they would by definition meet the broad requirements for vestibular migraine even though they actually have two separate medical conditions. The resulting incorrect diagnosis would then cause a delay in their true diagnosis and set them on a path for unnecessary or ineffective treatment, often at the cost of significant time and financial burden.

Over the past two decades a significant amount of research has been directed at vestibular migraine. This in turn led to a wealth of new information that allowed researchers to begin to separate out the symptoms of vestibular migraine from the many other medical conditions that present similarly. Eventually, this information was formed into what became the diagnostic criteria for vestibular migraine. To help ensure that truly sick vestibular migraine patients were not incorrectly excluded, as well as ensuring that those who do not have vestibular migraine were indeed excluded from diagnosis, the Bárány society in 2012 established two categories for vestibular migraine – vestibular migraine and *probable* vestibular migraine[55]. This establishment of diagnostic guidelines was a major step for vestibular migraine and allows for a more consistent and wider understanding of the condition.

In defining the diagnosis of a vestibular migraine, it can best be summed up through a direct quote from their published guidelines[55]:

[t]he diagnosis of vestibular migraine is based on recurrent vestibular symptoms, a history of migraine, a temporal association between vestibular symptoms and migraine symptoms and exclusion of other causes of vestibular symptoms. Symptoms that qualify for a diagnosis of vestibular migraine include various types of vertigo as well as head motion-induced dizziness with nausea. Symptoms must be of moderate or severe intensity. Duration of acute episodes is limited to a window of between 5 minutes and 72 hours.

The actual wording of the diagnostic criteria is much more involved and we'll next outline these criteria as established by the Bárány society. As mentioned, the society has established two categories – 'vestibular migraine' and 'probable vestibular migraine', with separate diagnostic criteria for each.

For a diagnosis of vestibular migraine, several criteria must be met, which include[55]:

A. A minimum of 5 episodes with vestibular symptoms of moderate or severe intensity that last 5 minutes to 72 hours

B. A current or previous history of migraine with or without the presence of aura as outlined by the International Classification of Headache Disorders (ICHD)

C. One or more symptoms of migraine during at least 50% of the vestibular episodes
   a. Headache with at least two of the following characteristics: having a one-sided location, a pulsating effect, moderate

to severe pain intensity, aggravation by routine physical activity
   b. Presence of photophobia and phonophobia
   c. Visual aura
D. Symptoms that are not better accounted for by another vestibular or ICHD diagnosis

Probable vestibular migraine has a similar classification despite fewer diagnostic requirements[55]. These requirements include:
   A. At least 5 episodes that have vestibular symptoms of moderate or severe intensity and last 5 min to 72 hours
   B. Having only one of the criteria B and C for vestibular migraine fulfilled (migraine history *or* migraine features during the episode)
   C. Symptoms that are not better accounted for by another vestibular or ICHD diagnosis

This definition of vestibular migraine is important as it not only fits the needs of the vestibular community, it is also accepted within the headache community as well[55]. This includes, for example, the Migraine Classification subcommittee of the International Headache Society.

Testing for vestibular migraine

Much like other vertigo-related conditions such as Ménière's disease, there are no specific biomarkers for vestibular migraine. In other words, a blood test or biopsy will not reveal whether an individual has vestibular migraine. Therefore, diagnosis must rely more on information provided by the patients such as symptoms and family history. With enough detail provided by the patient, a medical professional can often arrive at the proper diagnosis; however, this highlights the importance of accurate descriptions, timeframes, and duration of the array of symptoms experienced by a patient. For example, one barrier to providing an accurate medical history is the improper description of the type of vertigo, particularly that patients don't always separate rotational or positional vertigo from dizziness or disequilibrium[93].

There are some inner-ear tests that can be performed which do provide valuable information towards a diagnosis of vestibular migraine. For example, up to one in five vestibular migraine patients – including children – exhibit a suppressed response to what is known as the caloric stimulation test[88]. This test evokes a particular eye movement when cool or warm air is gently blown into the ear canal. Separately, controlled movement of the eye can be altered in some vestibular migraine patients[70]. Other vestibular-based tests reveal unique findings in some vestibular migraine patients, but the details of those results will not be outlined here. It is important to note, though, that the percent of patients with vestibular migraine reported to have abnormal findings in response to vestibular testing is not consistently high; rather, the percent of patients with positive results for a particular test often hover in the 25-50% range[88]. This indicates that not all vestibular migraine patients will have test results consistent with vestibular migraine findings. To counter this issue, a battery of tests can often reveal trends in results that can allow medical professionals to arrive at a likely diagnosis.

The relatively low amount of information that can be derived from these vestibular tests is why it is key that you as a sufferer provide a thorough medical history along with a highly detailed list of symptoms and triggers to your medical provider.

Similarity to other conditions

One of the challenges in diagnosing vestibular migraine is that the condition is very similar in symptoms to Ménière's disease as well as BPPV (see Chapter 8). All conditions produce episodes of sudden vertigo, but there are also distinct differences that do exist between these conditions. It is usually the application of each condition's diagnostic criteria that separates them from vestibular migraine and allows for a tailored treatment plan.

There are several examples of similar symptoms between multiple vestibular disorders. Obviously, vestibular migraine, BPPV and Ménière's disease all involve some degree of vertigo and/or vestibular-related symptoms. However, migraine headaches, photophobia, and auras have been reported with both Ménière's disease and vestibular migraines[20, 118]. And patients with BPPV suffer migraines much like vestibular migraine patients do[1, 119]. Moreover, persistent symptoms like dizziness or unsteadiness are commonly reported in almost all patients affected by vestibular migraine, BPPV, and Ménière's disease.

Despite many similarities between these vestibular-related conditions, there are also significant differences. For example, Ménière's disease typically involves some degree of hearing loss, particularly at the lower-frequencies[92, 120]. Vestibular migraine patients may experience some inner-ear involvement such as fluctuating hearing loss, tinnitus, or pressure in the ear, but there is typically very minimal hearing loss[55]. Furthermore, Ménière's attacks typically last from 20 minutes to 12 hours[120] while vestibular migraine attacks can last for two days[67, 120]. Age can also be a determinant, as vestibular migraine can occur with some frequency in adolescents[112] while Ménière's and BPPV typically happen in an older population[121, 122]. Despite these differences, it is important that patients provide as much detail about their illness as possible. Such detail can often be accomplished through the use of a daily activity log.

While it is certainly possible that a vestibular patient has a particular condition that mimics another, it has also been shown that patients can have multiple disorders such as vestibular migraine *and* Ménière's disease. One study that looked at nearly 150 patients with vestibular migraine found that one-fourth of those patients also had Ménière's disease[123]. Additionally, half of those Ménière's patients had headache, contributing to the belief that the underlying issues triggering both vestibular migraine and Ménière's disease likely have some commonalities[102]. Separately, we have discussed in an earlier chapter that vestibular migraine patients may experience vertigo when the head is in certain positions. This positional vertigo is similar to a common factor of BPPV, where certain head positions can trigger bouts of vertigo.

Conclusion

Diagnosis of vestibular migraine has been a work in progress for several decades. The development of specific diagnostic criteria has certainly aided medical professionals in diagnosis, but other medical conditions which closely match the symptoms of vestibular migraine can still impede proper diagnosis. Furthermore, patients may have separate conditions such as BPPV and migraine that are also present in vestibular migraine, but merely overlap rather than have a direct association with each other. It is essential that vestibular migraine patients provide a thorough history of symptoms and events to their medical professional so that relevant symptoms can be assessed and so that targeted treatment can be initiated.

Chapter 6: My Story

ITʹS HARD TO IMAGINE THE POWER that the vestibular system maintains over us. Well, itʹs hard to imagine until yours has started to malfunction, anyway. Iʹve been there. Iʹve also had a point where I had not only what I would classify as a migraine, but also a period during which I had some degree of constant and continuous headache for over a year. I wrote this chapter to outline for you as a migraine sufferer that I understand what youʹre going through. Iʹve had my own inner-ear issues, and as a result I not only have compassion for what youʹre dealing with but also a great deal of respect for the fact that you are able to handle it. It takes immense effort and drive to put up with the constant unsteadiness, dizziness, vertigo, attacks, and migraine that you live with every day, and I will be the first to say that no one – and I mean no one – can understand the overpowering effects of a vestibular migraine attack unless theyʹve had one. Nor can they grasp an idea of the constant battles you face even in between your attacks. This chapter, outlining my own experience, likely pales in response to what many of you live with every day, as I have never officially been diagnosed with vestibular migraine even though I had a time period where I experienced many of the same symptoms. Hopefully you will see that you are not alone in what you are dealing with, and that help – and success – is certainly possible.

As I said, I've experienced multiple inner-ear conditions in my lifetime, including both BPPV and Ménière's disease. And, I live every day with tinnitus. In the interest of full disclosure, I have no issue saying again that I myself have never been diagnosed with vestibular migraine. So, you might ask, why would I write a book on vestibular migraine if I've never even had it? Truth be told, that answer has multiple components. First and foremost, there are several events that I have dealt with in prior years that are more representative of vestibular migraine than my other, diagnosed conditions. Second, I don't feel that there are any *good* books out there on the topic of vestibular migraine that are written for patients. There are certainly books out there, but I don't think that they are written in a way that helps educate patients. They're either too technical in nature or they're trying to sell a product. And neither of those fit my goal of what I want to accomplish with this book. My third reason for writing this book is that I have written several other books covering inner-ear conditions, and quite frankly, it's very satisfying to hear patients of those conditions tell me that they enjoyed and benefitted from my books. Therefore, based on that feedback, I wanted to take on this book as well, with the intent of not only learning more about the condition but also serving to provide you a viable resource guide specific to vestibular migraine.

My initial experience with the 'joy' of vestibular conditions was when I dealt with BPPV after taking an accidental knee to my head back in 2002. After a few months of dealing with vertigo every time I tilted my head back, I eventually found complete relief through the miracle of the Epley maneuvers. I thought that my time with dizziness was done, but little did I know that my days with BPPV was just the beginning of a long and certainly troubling, hand-in-hand journey with my middle ear.

Though I don't remember the exact date, I certainly remember that fateful morning back in the early 2000's. I woke up around 6am in the middle of a raging thunderstorm. As I got out of bed in order to make my way to the shower, I noticed suddenly that my balance was off. *Way* off. I stepped closer to my bedroom wall in order to use it to brace myself up. A range of thoughts raced through my mind as a result of the strange effects I was feeling. Was my BPPV back? Did I have a stroke? A sudden ear infection? Was some change in barometric pressure from the storm affecting my balance? Despite the unexplained imbalance, I recognized that it wasn't really the same as the vertigo I had experienced during my BPPV days. Rather, it was a combination of dizziness and unsteadiness. My initial intent was that I might be able to walk it off – a sort of 'pushing through it', if you might, to the point that my body would figure out how to overcome whatever it was that was out of whack just enough to cause my unsteadiness. But this plan, though simple in theory, was quickly overruled by an inability to maintain my balance without leaving my hands against the walls as I walked down even a short hallway. As I failed to make any significant improvement with each passing minute, my mind started racing. Could I go to work? Is this permanent?

Eventually I realized that walking was my biggest problem - if I stayed seated I didn't seem to have much of an issue. Therefore I carefully got dressed and prepared to head to work. At that point I had a sudden thought – maybe it is really just my BPPV making a return. Perhaps I had rolled over in bed just precisely enough to cause some otoliths to escape their vestibular home. If so, a quick canalith repositioning should improve my situation. At the time, canalith repositioning was relatively new in the medical world. I'd had it done to fix my own BPPV just a year or two earlier, and at the time it required a soft neck brace and maintaining a vertical head position for 48 hours (though now, neither the brace nor maintaining head position are required). As I laid down and put myself through the maneuvers, I was hopeful for a quick fix. About a minute later, I stood up. My hopes were dashed with the first unsteady sway I felt.

My acceptance grew that I would just be dizzy for a while, and maybe this was some sort of congestion or ear-infection problem that would work itself out. I drove to work carefully, the dizziness seemingly subdued somewhat compared to the issues I had earlier felt when walking. As the day progressed, the dizziness and imbalance failed to dissipate. Unfortunately it had also triggered faint hints of nausea, even though those hints never turned into actual vomiting.

This onset of additional symptoms gave me suspicion as to another potential cause for my dizziness, which in turn allowed me to develop yet another suspected fix for this new ailment. In my profession at that time I had been making several long bus trips during the winter months. I had always been a bit prone to motion sickness since my youth, and on some of these recent bus trips I had been developing a bit of motion sickness. So, I had talked to my physician about some medication that might help. He prescribed me phenergan at the time, which did an amazing job of halting the motion sickness as well as helping me sleep in a vehicle. Given this past success, I thought that my current dizziness situation may be some sort of leftover motion-sickness-related condition. If so, a dose of phenergan may be just what I need to get me back to normal.

One good thing about your friend also being your physician is that you can make a direct call to their cell phone when you need their quick attention. An hour later, I had phenergan in my hand. 20 minutes after taking a dose – the usual timeframe for suppression of any motion sickness – I noticed no difference. 30 minutes later I felt sleepy, but as dizzy as ever. Another well-intentioned plan was foiled.

When you have such an over-powering condition as one that is associated with the vestibular system, it can be difficult to forget that it's there. Other conditions, perhaps even a few devastating ones, manifest themselves under the surface, at times never making their presence known until it's time for a checkup or a procedure. Vestibular conditions are not this way. You are reminded of them all the time. Constantly. Because you move all the time, even if it's just turning your head side-to-side.

And so this became my routine – constantly being reminded that something was wrong, something that caused me unsteadiness and dizziness all the time. And still, this came across as a different type of dizziness than that which occurred as a result of my BPPV. When going through my BPPV phase I typically had forceful vertigo for about 15 seconds when tilting my head back, but I was relatively fine when not tilting my head back. This dizziness, however, did not let up. But at the same time, I was not experiencing any vertigo like I was with BPPV.

For a while, the dizziness and unsteadiness were significant, but I could manage them. Riding in a car could get me a little nauseous at times, but I was used to that as since a little kid I had always been the one that got carsick before everyone else. Within a week or so I had adapted to this new annoyance, and just resigned myself to doing periodic mental checks to see if there was any improvement. Despite being annoying, I had to admit and accept that the dizziness and unsteadiness was tolerable.

But then, one afternoon at work, I had a new issue – a headache. I've had headaches in my life, but this one was different. It was on the top of my head, just a few inches back from my forehead. It increased in intensity within two specific spots, almost as if two pointed, 10-pound weights were sitting on each side of a line that separated my skull into left and right sides. As the intensity of this headache increased, I started to feel a bit uncomfortable about being unable to drive if it worsened much more. Therefore I did something I've rarely had to do – I went home sick.

Once home, I crawled into bed as the headache continued to worsen. Even applying an ice bag directly to the area did nothing to reduce the pain. My thoughts turned toward thinking *so this is what a migraine feels like!* I'd heard of migraines, and from my understanding of them I had a pretty good idea of what 'intense' and 'painful' must mean. In my mind, what I was experiencing at that moment had to be of a level that qualified it as a migraine. Even though I consider myself a rather tough person, the headache was becoming overpowering. Eventually, I decided that the small bit of sleepiness I was also feeling might open me up to take a quick nap. If I could sleep, maybe I would be able to wake up and find out that it's all better. If it wasn't better, though, I decided that for the first time in my life I would have to make an emergency room trip.

As I laid there in bed, I started to believe that I just wasn't going to fall asleep. The pain of the headache was going to keep me up for a long, long time. Or so I thought, anyway. The next thing I knew, I had been asleep for an hour. And suddenly, a quick self-check revealed that my headache was *gone*. Those two powerfully painful spots had disappeared, leaving me with nothing but a very minor, almost residual-type headache that I pretty much dismissed as an after-effect of the powerful 'migraine' that I had just dealt with. Given that it was my first experience with such an overpowering headache, I was almost thankful to just be dealing with the minor, leftover effects that I now felt.

In the following days, though, I realized that something else was different along with my new companions named unsteadiness and dizziness. That small lingering headache that I had experienced continued to linger. Every day. It would fluctuate from slightly painful to annoying, although it never reached the level of the original migraine. Over time, as the days turned to weeks, I noticed that the headache was still there, joining in with my ongoing balance and dizziness issues. And if one day I felt that it was diminished – which gave me hope that it was improving – I was reminded the next day that it was still present, often making that presence known with a vengeance.

I also noticed something else unique about my headaches. They almost always worsened through the morning, sometimes reaching a tolerable peak and other times becoming somewhat painful, so much that they were clearly a distraction. Then during the summer months I made a new discovery. My work hours were diminished during the summers, and I was often able to head home by noon, if not earlier. Given the increased fatigue I would feel in the afternoons since developing this constant headache, I would often get sleepy. This led me to take an afternoon nap, and I soon noticed that even though the headache increased in intensity during the day, it would always be significantly improved once I woke up from even a brief nap. It wasn't a coincidence resulting from me taking a nap at the point the headache went away on its own, for if I couldn't get in a nap, the headache would stay with me all day. It was weird, actually. If I tried to push through and wait for improvement, it never came. But if I took a quick nap, the headache would always go from a level '7' or so down to a level '3'. Though the obvious question might be *why not just take a nap each time*, the answer is that finding a time or location for a nap wasn't always feasible due to work and other obligations. But one thing was certain – the headaches were never as severe as that first one. And for that, I was thankful.

Over time, I noticed that the headache would have certain aspects that repeated randomly over time. One day it was low on my skull, almost in my neck. The next day it would be a band across my forehead. Other days it was like it was 'behind' my face, or along the side of my head. Through trial and error, I eventually found that one medication actually seemed to help during those times that I couldn't take a nap – an over-the-counter pill that contained a combination of acetaminophen, caffeine, and aspirin. To help prevent my becoming reliant upon it through daily use, I tried to use it only during the 'bad' headaches. But it made enough of a difference that I eventually ended up holding on to several bottles – one for home, one for work, and one kept in my car. The medicine certainly reduced the severity of the headache even though it never fully removed the presence of the headache itself. And try as I might, I couldn't determine any pattern or triggers for the headache – just that it was always there in some form, and always worsening as the day progressed. I still wanted to believe that the headaches were tied to my earlier BPPV events, but putting my head in the same position as what used to trigger my BPPV elicited no effect. And performing the Epley maneuvers resulted in no improvement or change in my dizziness, so the evidence indicated that it was something else causing these ongoing issues. And the worst part was that I had no idea what it was.

For most people there is a fine line between having a particular medical issue and actually going to get it looked at. For me, mine wasn't a fine line but rather a very thick, almost uncrossable line. My education is based in the medical field, and for years I had spent my efforts taking care of the medical problems that others have. So, since the unsteadiness I was still experiencing wasn't exactly debilitating and because I was able to keep my headaches in check with the medication, I felt it was best to press on and wait for there to be some degree of improvement.

Eventually, though, other things started to happen that ultimately did push me to take further action. My right ear had been feeling 'full' all the time, similar to what you might experience when congested with a head cold. And that fullness was combined with a 'roaring' sound, similar (in a much louder way) to what you'd expect if you held a seashell up against your ear. As a result of these ongoing symptoms, my hearing in that ear had become significantly worse. My left ear, though, was fine; therefore I would always have to turn towards a speaker so that my left ear was closer. This began a phase of fear and then acceptance that I was about to lose all hearing in my right ear. Though perhaps only coincidence, my less-functioning right ear was also the ear affected by BPPV, so I secretly held out hope that there was a quick fix still awaiting my discovery.

Slowly I had begun to notice even more strange new things happening. My vision started to change, to the point where I now noticed that if I stared at a very small spot, my vision would shake in very tiny amounts. I also began to have small flashes appearing in my peripheral vision, almost like tiny glowing little suns with short tails that swam around in twisting circles like bright little yellow sperm cells. I also noticed 'trails' when my field of view passed over a bright light. If, for example, I were driving at night and there was a car in front of me, if I passed my eyes back and forth from one side of that car to another, I would see a trail of 20-30 little headlights that lessened in intensity the further away from the car that they were.

These compounding events finally led me to take action. My physician friend had moved 100 miles away, so I had switched to a new personal physician. Telling her my symptoms, she recommended an MRI which ultimately revealed nothing. She then felt that a referral to an ear, nose, and throat (ENT) physician would be the best line of attack. To this day, I remember clearly the face that the ENT made when listening to my symptoms. I would describe it as a mix between shocked, clueless, and a sort of *"what the hell?"* expression. To put it bluntly, it was clear to me that he had no idea what I was talking about. The only thing I learned from his cursory evaluation was that I did in fact have a deviated septum. That, and a recommendation that I should just try to 'relax'.

The ENT's lack of any findings, combined with my certainty that 'something' was wrong, led me to return to my audiologist for another evaluation. Despite her tests, the results showed that my BPPV was in no way recurring, so that hope was dashed. But the visit also pointed out that the hearing in my right ear was significantly worse than my left, and much worse than my appointment almost two years earlier during my BPPV diagnosis. I expected this finding, given the roaring sound that was now almost always present. Although she didn't have any answers for my situation, the audiologist gave me the name of a physician in nearby Houston to see if I felt that I wanted a higher-level opinion. My answer was a resounding 'yes'.

My next stop was a neurologist in Houston two hours away. While I wasn't exactly sure I'd walk away with an answer, I felt that I'd get something more than the confused look I was given at the ENT. It was December of 2003 now, and I was over a year into this misery. I just needed *something* to give me hope that there was an end in sight. During the visit, I was slightly encouraged by the fact that the physician saw "something" on my MRI and requested another MRI scan as a result. You might wonder why someone might be encouraged by such news, as what he saw could certainly be a tumor or some other devastating event, but by this time I just wanted an answer as to what was going on inside my skull. I'd had no improvement in my constant dizziness or headache, so any hint at a cause as to what could be triggering these ongoing issues would be welcome news. In other words, at least finding something on an MRI might lead me to begin targeted treatment.

Unfortunately, what I found out was that the mysterious little area on the MRI was nothing more than a blurry spot, and I was left with no new answers from the neurologist. I can't tell if it's more frustrating to be told you have a particular medical condition or to be told that they can't find anything wrong. If they tell you what you have, at least you can begin to solve the problem. If they can't tell you what's wrong, despite your obvious symptoms, you can't make any real progress towards fixing the problem and you are left with a tremendous feeling of hopelessness. And that's where I was at during this time. I had daily, ongoing symptoms of dizziness, imbalance, and a non-functioning ear, but could not find anyone who could tell me what was causing these issues. In my mind, I had to start to accept that I was going to have to live like this. Without any understanding of what was causing my symptoms, I certainly couldn't make progress toward treating the conditions.

And so that's what I did – I accepted that this is just how life was going to be. The next few years were filled with random degrees of intense headache, phases of imbalance, and a continuation of symptoms that even got mixed in with a few new ones like a real sensitivity to loud sounds. I continued on with the headache medicine as needed, but over time the symptoms either became more tolerable, or I just learned to deal with them better. For the next five or so years I gradually became able to function without interruption. But then I started having sudden, random bouts of vertigo for several years. Eventually, as the vertigo and a whole new set of symptoms arrived in addition to what I was dealing with already, I was eventually diagnosed with Ménière's disease. This led to a major set of lifestyle changes, and I was eventually able to effectively eliminate all of my symptoms – except tinnitus – thanks to a targeted treatment plan for Ménière's. The nystagmus, unsteadiness, plugged ear, and even attacks eventually stopped, and I now live effectively 100% normal short of a few random 'blips' every now and then. But the details of that story are told in another book.

What I finally rationalized just a few years ago was that my initial symptoms when waking up that fateful morning must have been some type of after-effects from a Ménière's attack that happened while I was asleep. For years I tried to figure out what would have caused that forceful, initial bout of dizziness, but I never had a clear cause outlined. Only after later experiencing other attacks did the symptoms make sense. So for now, I'll chalk up my years of early symptoms as being a by-product of an initial Ménière's-related event. But truth be told, I often wonder if those early bouts with dizziness and imbalance – coupled with the constant headache and vision issues – were in fact a form of vestibular migraine. Quite frankly, I may never know. But I will be the first to say that the experience has given me a strong and valuable insight into the life of a vestibular migraine sufferer.

Chapter 7: Treatment of Vestibular Migraine

I F YOU LISTEN CLOSELY ENOUGH you might soon find out that there are about as many recommended treatments and cures for vestibular migraine as there are stars in the sky. OK, that might be a *little* bit of an over-exaggeration, but if you spend any time on message boards, internet groups, or even just talk to a few random people about your condition, you'll quickly discover that there are many treatments that will no doubt 'fix' your illness. Unfortunately, these treatments are largely anecdotal in nature, which is to say that they are nothing more than a bit of information that someone heard, or perhaps something that they themselves tried and ultimately perceived some sort of benefit. Usually, the vast majority of these treatments are quite harmless in their design. But another issue is that many of these treatments are also nothing more than unproven sales pitches, even if they are everyday items you can find in your cabinet. This is not to say that they are all worthless or that there aren't some vestibular migraine patients who might experience an actual effect from trying many of the purported treatments. Rather, the desperation that some vestibular migraine patients can have after years of minimal to no improvement can make them easy victims for scams that can have significant financial impact. Therefore, the first portion of this chapter on treatments for vestibular migraine will focus on what is known as the scientific process, a method that the best, scientifically-backed treatments and studies have gone through. The purpose is to educate you the vestibular migraine patient on how to perform your own evaluation on the treatments (and research) you hear about in order to make an informed decision that is best for *your* health. To be clear, this section is not to criticize certain vestibular migraine treatments; rather, it is to help you recognize the process that should be used in evaluating treatment and success claims. I have included this scientific process material in another book about an inner-ear condition, and the feedback from readers was overwhelmingly positive that it helped make them a better-educated consumer and patient. Based on that feedback, I feel that it is equally important to share this material in a book about vestibular migraine.

The scientific process

Science is all about observations. If a researcher designs an experiment, he or she already has a predicted outcome more commonly known as the *hypothesis*. By observing what happens during an experiment, his or her hypothesis will be supported or rejected. In some cases, hypotheses are relatively simple, such as *if I flip a coin, it will reveal 'heads' 50% of the time.* There is pretty much a one-in-two chance that the coin will show 'heads', as there are only two sides to the coin. Therefore, your hypothesis is quite simple to prove, for if you drop the coin enough times, it's highly likely that heads or tails will occur 50% of the time.

One thing about good science is that it is never permitted to simply *assume.* You still have to test your hypothesis in order to see if you were indeed correct. After all, there may be some unknown, small factor that influences your experiment. What if, for example, someone handed you a pair of die that when rolled, came up as a "three" and "four" 84% of the time? Wouldn't that seem a little odd versus what you would predict? If so, your hypothesis of expecting completely random numbers over and over would be refuted. A little further investigation may reveal that the dice were rigged to come up as a total of "7". So even though you expected that a pair of dice would provide random pairs of numbers, you still have to test your prediction to ensure that there is not some unknown factor influencing the results.

As I mentioned, making predictions using coins or dice are quite simple examples. Things get much more complicated in terms of experiments and predictions when it comes to fields like medicine or psychology. If a researcher designs a drug with the intent for that drug to cure a specific condition, it is relatively simple in concept to design the drug molecule to fit and bind to a specific receptor in the body that should generate an action that the researcher intends. However, it is much more complicated to get that drug molecule to the area of the body it needs to be, or survive the digestive system, or stay in an active form long enough for it to bind to its receptor. In addition, researchers also have to be able to predict any side-effects or unwanted conditions that may result from that drug; otherwise, even if a drug performs its intended duty, too serious of side effects would ultimately prevent its use. Furthermore, they have to show that whatever positive and negative effects occur do in fact occur consistently across several individuals with that condition. It can be a frustrating and difficult process, but it is essential for establishing the 'truth' about the effects of a drug or treatment product.

Unfortunately, establishing all of these factors takes both time and money. A researcher typically has to obtain a grant in order to pay for the facilities, staff, and equipment to design their treatment (i.e. drug, machine, etc.) for a specific condition. On top of that, the researcher has to get approval from a board of experts before they are even allowed to begin their experiment, an often drawn-out process that serves to ensure that what the researcher is proposing is both ethical and necessary. And if they reveal legitimate results – sometimes only in a test tube – they have to be able to show that their results can be replicated (i.e. repeated) across a wide variety of individuals of various backgrounds and health statuses, yet another drawn-out process. Once that occurs and there is a clear and safe benefit in using the drug or product, the researcher will most likely be able to start marketing his or her product. When done properly, this process can take years.

In light of the effort required to develop and test a potential treatment effectively, many individuals and companies have decided that it's much simpler to just forego all of the bureaucratic 'nonsense' and post some treatment online that they believe is effective. The problem in doing so is that there often lacks real evidence that the treatment actually works. And, the person selling the treatment often knows that the product has no proof – especially when there is a potential financial gain in store for them if they can just convince enough people to buy the product.

Testing on subjects

In order to outline why it is important that products work across groups of people rather than just a single person, we need to look at what is commonly referred to as a *subject*, or an individual involved in experimental testing.

Humans are very similar but very different from each other. Stand two individuals of the same gender, height, and weight next to each other and you might say that they are very similar. But, if you investigate deeper into what you can't see, you might find that one is allergic to a substance, or has high blood pressure, or maybe has an autoimmune disorder. In other words, looking at their outward appearance tells you nothing about particular details that you can't see, such as an underlying medical condition. So, what may be beneficial or safe for one of them might not be the case for both. However, if a researcher can show that a treatment works for *many* – even though it may not work for 'everyone' – it can be cause for getting that treatment approved and on the market.

In medicine, when something applies to a single entity, such as a person, location, or event, it is referred to as a *case*. For example, a flu outbreak at a school after a student returns from a trip would be specific to that school, and is not particularly relevant to *all* schools. Therefore, that particular flu outbreak could be considered a case for that school. Similarly, if a patient is allergic to, say bacon, that would make his or her situation a case specific to him or her rather than an expected reaction for everyone, as the vast majority of people are not allergic to bacon. Medical treatments apply similarly – if something works for one single patient, it doesn't necessarily mean that it is an effective treatment. Likewise, if one person cannot use a treatment due to an allergy or some other situation, it does not mean that 'all' individuals should not use the treatment. But, if a treatment works for many people in a variety of situations (i.e. a "pool" of individuals), it is much more likely that the treatment truly works.

When it comes to vestibular migraine treatments and 'cures', there is no shortage of unique options available online. Many of these treatments have not only failed to go through the experimental design process as described earlier, but you will also find little evidence of consistent effects. Product descriptions may highlight a testimonial or two, but the question you as the patient and consumer have to ask yourself is whether that testimonial is valid and whether that positive comment is worth you purchasing the product. After all, it's no secret that people can get paid to make positive comments about a product.

To outline how a useless product can seem to some consumers to be a miracle cure, we can use the example of an old phone scam that perfectly outlines how people can fall for false promises. Say you are a swindler and you are needing some cash. You call 40 people, 20 to whom you tout a new, 'hot' stock "A" and 20 to whom you tout stock "B". Stock A ends up doing poorly, so you never call back that group. But stock "B" does well, so you call back those people and say "see, I *told* you it would do well!". Knowing that your potential victims aren't quite sold on your service, you then tell half of those remaining people to buy stock "C", and half to buy stock "D". But only stock "D" ends up doing well. Therefore, you quickly call back the people you told about stock "D", bragging about your skills as a stock genius and asking if they are finally ready to invest. Given what appeared to be your two hot recommendations, many in the group hand over money to you to invest for them. What the people in that group don't know is that 30 of your 40 original phone calls went unreturned due to a lack of performance. Consequently, they are quick to hand you their money to invest – after which you skip town, never to be seen again.

Internet-based vestibular migraine treatment options can work similarly. Sure, a person can tout the effects of a treatment, but how many did the treatment *not* work well for? If a $10 treatment works on 20 people but does not work on 80, is that a financial risk? Not really, and depending on the potential harm (hopefully there is none) it may be worth trying if nothing else has worked for a patient. But, what if that rarely successful treatment is a series of steps that take a month to complete, costs $400, and has the same 20% success rate? You might be a bit hesitant to partake in such a treatment, and you certainly should be skeptical.

When skepticism arises, your next step should be to simply investigate the claims made. Who made the claim? If the company is touting their own product or performed their own research on their own manufactured product, red flags – a lot of them – should be raised. If the product was tested independently, such as by a researcher who has no ties to the company, it can greatly improve the validity of the product claims. But putting a product through the testing phase costs money, and it is often much easier to just market the product to desperate people and convince them that it works. Maybe even pay some consumers to write the aforementioned favorable testimonial which will most likely make it onto the manufacturer's website. As potential customers look through the website, a bunch of positive reviews makes it tempting to purchase the product. But, isn't that really what effective marketing is supposed to do – convince you to buy a product? As the price you are willing to pay increases, you as the consumer and patient have to carefully decide if the product is worth the risk. And having solid information about how the product was tested can play an important role in your decision.

True effects vs coincidence

Along the same lines of establishing whether a product works on a single patient or is effective across a range of patients, it is also important to evaluate the facts about the treatment's reported effects. For example, say a person goes to a rock concert full of loud, booming speakers, and later that night has a good bit of ringing in his ear. A friend gives him an oil to put in his ear, and when he wakes up, the ringing is greatly diminished. The second day after the rock concert, and after a little bit more oil was applied, the ringing disappeared. Does that mean that the oil fixed his tinnitus? Or could it be that he simply didn't have the true chronic-type tinnitus that many individuals suffer from, and therefore it went away on its own?

Given the circumstances, it's highly likely that the rock concert caused temporary tinnitus that resolved itself in a few hours. Therefore the oil had no real effect at all; rather, it was just pure coincidence that the application of the oil coincided with the natural reduction in tinnitus. But what do you think might happen when a few years later that same person runs into a colleague who is complaining of constant ringing in her ear for the past six weeks? There's little doubt that he'll end up touting the effects of the oil that he is certain stopped his own tinnitus. And given the long-term status of her tinnitus, she'll probably want to give it a try.

This scenario outlines the classic situation where a misinterpretation of effects leads to belief in a treatment that doesn't really work. Unfortunately, with chronic conditions such as vestibular migraine that can create patients who are desperate for relief, there are individuals that capitalize on this desperation in order to sell treatments that have no realistic chance of working. I often see it myself online, and that is the main reason for my adding this 'introduction to research' to the chapter – to make you as a patient and consumer more aware. So, let's look a little deeper into what you should be assessing when it comes to a vestibular migraine treatment.

Designing experiments

When science looks for a new treatment, it applies the treatment to one group (the experimental group) and no treatment to another identical group (the control group). Then, differences are evaluated between the groups, with the experimental group typically expected to have a favorable outcome. For example, if there was a belief that low iron intake caused vestibular migraine, it could be *tested* by designing an appropriate experiment. The two groups would be equally comprised of individuals of similar gender and age as well as both duration and severity of vestibular migraine. In other words, you wouldn't want to apply the new treatment to a group of, say, females, and then use all males in the control group. Rather, you want consistency in the makeup of the subjects between the two groups. Therefore, you would establish each group so that they consist of similar individuals (e.g. comparable vestibular migraine duration, gender, age, etc.). Then, for the experiment you would add the iron supplements to a meal for the experimental group while supplying the same meal to the control group, but without the added iron supplement. As long as everything else stays the same, any consistent results occurring in the experimental group (such as an improvement in the majority of the group's vestibular migraine symptoms after consuming the additional iron) should be expected to be due to the treatment, and not random coincidence. If there is no improvement in the experimental group after the additional iron intake, it could be determined that the treatment of iron supplementation has no effect.

We discussed how the makeup of the experiment and control group is important. If, as mentioned, the groups are not made of similar individuals, you would effectively be comparing apples to oranges and therefore, any results you obtain from the experiment would have no real validity. Besides physical makeup such as age and gender, similarity in symptoms between groups is important as well. For example, if you had one group that reported having mild migraine and vertigo symptoms for six months and another group had debilitating vestibular migraine for at least ten years, keeping them separated into individual experimental and control groups would result in a major study design flaw. However, if you *mixed* the groups so that some people with short-term and others with long-term symptoms and severity were in the same group, that would be acceptable as it creates a "pool' of subjects of similar conditions between the experimental and control groups.

It is also strongly recommended that the groups are comprised of enough people to capture the possible variations in the condition (i.e. vestibular migraine) that could affect the results. Do the groups capture all severities of vestibular migraine, or just a specific one or two types? Is the long-term group all taking a certain medication? Have they had a certain procedure? If so, these particular situations become *confounders* if they can influence the experiment's results. Say, for example, that ¾ of the people in the aforementioned experimental group were also taking a 'headache supplement' that interfered with iron metabolism. If those same people then took the iron supplement, the iron would have no chance to exert its potential effects on vestibular migraine. Therefore, the experiment's results may end up showing that only some of the people in the experimental group had an improvement in their vestibular migraine symptoms after taking an iron supplement. However, if those same people were also the ones that were *not* taking the headache supplement, it would make the experiment's results look as though the iron was not very effective when in fact the iron was being prevented from working in some people in the experimental group because they were taking the headache supplement. Therefore, study design is vital and must include aspects such as ensuring that the group's subjects are properly selected and screened, and confounding factors (such as some subjects taking a certain headache supplement) are controlled.

This may seem like a lot of detail for a vestibular migraine patient to be worried about, but truth be told, these concepts should be a key factor in whether that consumer elects to try out a particular treatment. And if a company is not willing to discuss how they arrived at their marketing claims such as *"reduced headache severity by 50%"*, it should immediately raise questions for anyone considering the treatment. For example, questions should be raised such as "Reduced in what population?" "How long was the treatment given?" "Did they have any other treatments or do anything else simultaneously?" "How and when was headache severity measured?" The more questions that can be answered legitimately, the more credibility the product gains.

There are certainly times when a treatment may only be tested and shown successful on a particular type of vestibular migraine patient such as females, or only when vertigo is present with a migraine, and that limited evidence is perfectly acceptable if the product is marketed as such. In those cases, it is fine to report the findings as long as the success is also reported to be *limited* to that particular population. Remember – assuming is not permitted when it comes to 'assuming' that a treatment reported in one group will apply similarly to another. In other words, if a treatment has not been tested on a particular type of vestibular migraine patient, it cannot be assumed that the treatment will work until that factor is addressed using a reputable scientific study. So, if a treatment is shown to reduce the incidence of vertigo attacks in postmenopausal vestibular migraine females, it cannot be assumed that the product will also work equally well in males until that has been shown with a proper experiment.

What is all of this saying? Simple – it is recommended that you strive to look for vestibular migraine treatments that have gone through the rigor of scientific testing if you're going to spend money on the treatment. There is actually much, much more that we could discuss regarding the scientific process and how it applies to vestibular migraine treatment, as we have just skimmed the surface. But, what we have discussed should help you to ask questions and read with more detail the evidence behind treatments that you encounter.

If there is no clear evidence or indication of a treatment's proof, I strongly suggest that you look elsewhere. At the same time, I am cognizant that there is no cure yet for vestibular migraine and as such, the cure remains 'out there' somewhere. If you look at how far we've progressed in our understanding of vestibular migraine over the past 30 years, it's clear that we have made significant progress. And as we continue to eliminate ineffective treatments, we strengthen the pool of effective options while also expanding our search into promising new areas. When considering an alternative treatment for your own vestibular migraine, consider the financial cost, the physical risk including side effects, and the evidence that exists for the treatment. The degree of proof that is required in order to use a particular treatment is ultimately left up to you.

Summarizing the scientific process

You may have been wondering if we were ever going to get to the part about treating vestibular migraine. The answer is certainly 'yes', but I wanted to include the previous material because it is important to me as an author that you understand how to wade through the vast amount of information that you will be presented with specific to treatment of vestibular migraine. As a former researcher, I am immediately skeptical of any claim presented as anecdotal (i.e. personal experience) rather than based in the scientific process; that is just the effect of my years of research-based training and it is not exactly right or wrong as a belief. To a vestibular migraine sufferer, though, living with the misery of an attack often leads them to try *anything* regardless of the purported benefits. And in many cases this can be ok as long as it doesn't cause physical or financial harm to you. But it can also lead to wasted time and false hope if you're not careful, and false hope often leads to repeated bouts of disappointment and/or depression as yet another hopeful cure falls flat. So, take the information you learned in this first part of the chapter and always be sure to perform your own level of evaluation of a treatment's effectiveness. If you read a claim online, look for the sources or research used to establish that claim. If you are told of a treatment that can help, ask what it is about the product that works, as well as how it works better than other available options. Being diligent about these claims can help ensure that you are making valuable progress toward a beneficial treatment that can help reduce your own symptoms.

Treatment for Vestibular Migraine

When it comes to treatment, there both "are" a lot of treatments for vestibular migraine and there equally "aren't" a lot of treatments. The reason I say this is because vestibular migraine is relatively new in the disease world and we just don't know much about it yet. In fact, as recently as 2015 only one double-blinded study had been conducted on vestibular migraine treatment[1]. As a result, we don't have a lot of effective treatments because science hasn't yet figured out what tissue or area of the body to target. Instead, vestibular migraine patients are often limited to treatments based on expert opinion[66], and much of the recommended care for vestibular migraine focuses on treatment guidelines for the headache associated with migraine[1]. So yes, you could say that there are many treatments out there, but the fact is that there just aren't very many true treatments that have a beneficial effect for vestibular migraine.

When I say *true* treatments, I am talking about those treatments which have been investigated using an experimental design such as what we talked about earlier in this chapter. I could easily say we will discuss *all* treatments for vestibular migraine, but the fact is that doing so would literally take volumes of books. This is simply due to the fact that there are probably *thousands* of 'treatments' out there. When you look at pharmaceutical, psychological, homeopathic, naturopathic, herbs, supplements, manual therapy, and even narcotic-derived (e.g. cannabidiol, or "CBD" oil), the options can be quite overwhelming in terms of separating out what has actually been shown to work even somewhat consistently versus what a person has stated worked for them (i.e. a single case). Therefore, in this chapter we will focus predominantly on treatments which the scientific community has investigated. Again, this is not to say that the wealth of at-home or homeopathic treatments are ineffective. Rather, it's just that there are so many of these treatments that it would be nearly impossible to adequately cover all of them in this chapter specific to the reported effectiveness of each.

Preventative measures

You've no doubt heard that prevention is the best medicine, and for a vestibular migraine sufferer who has been through an attack, it's almost a guarantee that they are willing to do most anything to prevent another attack from happening. Obviously, if there was one treatment, whether it be pharmaceutical, physical, or even psychological that actually worked well in preventing an attack, everyone would be using it. The problem is that there just isn't yet a clear and effective treatment that has consistent effects across vestibular migraine patients. Therefore, patients are pretty much limited to the typical preventative-type treatments such as getting adequate sleep, eating a healthy diet, and avoiding those known triggers (e.g. stress, certain foods, etc.)

that we discussed in an earlier chapter[124]. Unfortunately, avoiding triggers or getting a full night's sleep isn't always an option, and patients are often left with the subsequent consequences. But over time you can expect to become better at avoiding your triggers, which will hopefully help reduce the incidence of attacks. Furthermore, as one study pointed out, until better medications or treatments are made available to patients, our current best practice of employing migraine treatment may be the most effective method for treating vestibular migraine patients[125]. Much like what is often recommended for vestibular migraine, traditional migraine recommendations also include eating a balanced diet, engaging in exercise, and obtaining adequate sleep, along with recognizing and avoiding known triggers such as caffeine[126].

Alongside engaging in healthy activity and avoidance of triggers, the first recommended treatment for vestibular migraine is often thorough counseling[88]. This can be effective at outlining for the patient the migraine involvement (especially if headache itself is not initially evident) as well as helping to alleviate the patient's unnecessary fears of a more serious medical condition. In addition, counseling can help the patient better prepare for the necessary lifestyle adjustments needed to cope with the disease.

Pharmaceutical treatment

One of the first things that a vestibular migraine sufferer will be provided is some form of drug therapy. This is, of course, after having gone through the diagnostic test process in order to rule out everything else such as Ménière's, BPPV, stroke, etc. Some individuals argue that non-drug treatment (i.e. avoidance of triggers, adequate sleep, etc.) can be as effective as medication use[88], and prior research has shown that specific to migraines, relaxation techniques as well as biofeedback can be as effective as medication at treating migraine[127]. As we just discussed in the first portion of this chapter, though, the fact that relaxation and biofeedback have been shown effective for migraine treatment does not infer that it will be equally successful for vestibular migraine.

The next phase of treatment often involves implementation of drug therapy. Pharmaceutical use is typically divided into two phases – the acute phase, which involves that portion of vestibular migraine specific to the random attacks, and the preventative phase, which is focused on treating the patient in-between attacks with an intent of either lessening or preventing a future attack.

Before we continue, I want to take a moment to make clear just what a drug is. In the online vestibular migraine world, there are a lot of recommendations out there as to what people 'have done', or 'should try' in order to improve their symptoms. Oftentimes in discussion groups you will find that sufferers are recommended to take (or have benefitted from) a supplement such as an herb or a spice (e.g. garlic, capsaicin, etc.) in order to improve their symptoms. It must be made clear that supplements are not drugs and should not be considered as pharmaceutical treatment. Drugs are substances which induce physiological change within the body. They may block a receptor from causing an action (e.g. inhibit the transmission of pain) or perhaps stop the production of a substance such as a hormone. Supplements, on the other hand, add to what is already consumed in the diet. Therefore, taking a calcium supplement only gives your body more calcium – it is not designed to cause a change within the body. As such, taking garlic or some other herb falls under supplementation rather than drug/medication therapy. Generally, supplementation is considered much safer than drug therapy as there is no physiological change expected within the body. However, because of the vast range of supplements that exist, their use in the treatment of vestibular migraine will not be covered in detail in this book.

Part of the problem with medication use is that for many people their vertigo attacks are transient in nature such that they don't last a long time even without drug therapy. Furthermore, some patients experience spontaneous remission of their vestibular migraine symptoms, even without treatment[88]. Such improvement of symptoms even without treatment can make it difficult to determine the effects of treatment in some cases. For example, the drug zolmitriptan has been shown to be somewhat effective for treating acute vertigo in vestibular migraine patients, as one study showed that 38% of patients had improved vertigo two hours post-treatment compared to just 22% of the placebo (non-drug) group[128]. These results, however, help illustrate that even without receiving drug treatment (i.e. the placebo group), some patients' vertigo does improve on its own. This in turn complicates the true, potential benefit of the drug, as even though 16% of sufferers in the study did report improvement, it calls into question how many of those sufferers also experienced spontaneous improvement of symptoms.

As outlined by such a study, treatment effectiveness can be complicated in that any medication – especially oral medication – given to the patient also takes a while to get into their system where it can actually have a beneficial effect. So it can often be difficult to determine whether a patient simply got better on their own through the subsiding of their symptoms or if they indeed benefitted from the medication itself. This is particularly true of those medications designed to stop or reduce the severity of acute attacks. So unfortunately, there are not a lot of studies out there that have directly investigated certain medications' benefit at reducing, stopping, or preventing vestibular migraine attacks. Still, certain drugs have been shown to be quite effective. However, understand that the drugs we discuss next are prescription in nature and will therefore require approval from your treating physician. Physicians, especially those trained in disorders related to vertigo and migraine, will be well-versed on the effects of these drugs. Therefore the decision to use these prescription medications must result from a discussion between you and your physician – NOT from this book!

Largely because of the relationship between acute vestibular migraine and migraine itself, patients are often treated using migraine medication with the intent that the medication can also help reign in any vestibular symptoms[60]. For example, when researchers looked at the effect of the drug triptan on vertigo, they determined that the reported benefits were actually due to the drug's ability to improve headache[129]. Furthermore, triptan has also been shown to positively influence motion sickness in migraine patients[130]. Almotriptan was shown to resolve vertigo within one hour in 55% of patients diagnosed with vestibular migraine[131]. In addition, 28% of patients reported a greater than 50% reduction in vertigo, while just 16% declared less than a 50% reduction in vertigo. Sumatriptan was shown in one study of 53 patients to be highly effective for reducing headache and moderately effective for reducing vertigo[129]. This same study reported that beta blockers, tricyclic antidepressants, methylsergide, valproic acid, and cyproheptadine were basically ineffective at treating vertigo.

Other vestibular migraine drugs can include those in the calcium-channel-blocking group such as flunarizine and cinnarizine[60] in addition to drug classes that include antiepileptics and antidepressants, all of which have mixed effects in treating vestibular migraine. Vestibular suppressants such as promethazine and meclizine have also been suggested[132] as well as dimenhydrinate[77].

Preventative drug treatment for vestibular migraine has similar mixed results as the acute drugs. Acetazolamide resulted in a reduced frequency of attacks, but six patients had to drop out of the study due to significant side effects of the drug and almost 9 in 10 patients reported adverse effects such as tingling in the extremities[133]. To a patient suffering from vestibular migraine, it can often be a difficult tradeoff between continuing to have vertigo attacks or taking a medication yet also putting up with the side effects of a drug. But you can imagine that if 1/10th of patients dropped out of a study due to negative side effects, the attack-reducing benefits of a drug must not have been worth the side effects for them. Similarly, cinnarizine is a calcium-channel blocker that has been found to reduce attack frequency as well as headache duration and intensity, but patients also reported weight gain, drowsiness, and blurry vision as side effects[134]. When combined with menhydrinate, cinnarizine was shown to reduce both vertigo and headache frequency by over 50% compared to lifestyle modification only, which also decreased the frequency but to a lesser degree[135].

Flunarizine was found to reduce vertigo symptoms compared to those who did not receive the drug, but it had no effect on headache frequency or severity[136]. Other studies with flunarizine found that 2/3 of patients reported an improvement in vestibular symptoms[104] and that it provided a significant improvement in symptoms[137]. However, flunarizine is a drug historically known to have significant side effects[138]. Separately, lamotrigine has been shown to reduce the frequency of vertigo as well, though it had no real effect on headache frequency[139].

Propranolol and venlafaxine both decreased the number of vertigo attacks over a four-month period, and venlafaxine also decreased the symptoms of depression[140]. Furthermore, another study found that propranolol improved vestibular symptoms in almost three out of four patients[104]. Six months of topiramate dropped the mean frequency of vertigo attacks from 5.5 to 1 in patients along with a significant decrease in the number of monthly headaches. In addition, vertigo severity decreased by 75%, with a 50% reduction in headache severity[141]. Unfortunately, this rather effective drug was found to have significant side effects that resulted in several participants dropping out.

Although there is some favorable evidence indicating that pharmaceutical treatment can be beneficial for improving vestibular migraine symptoms, recent research has suggested that there are no recommendations for drug use in the *prevention* of vestibular migraine[142]. This decision was led in part by the degree of side effects of many drugs as well as the lack of consistent benefit from available drugs. This belief, however, is not universally supported in the vestibular migraine world. Others have recommended that drug therapy can be effective but should be re-evaluated after three months[88]. During this time period, a goal targeted at a reduction in attacks of about 50-70% should be established. Therefore, it is important for patients to keep a daily log of not only their triggers but also their attack frequency in order to help their physician determine whether their treatments are effective.

One of the hindrances of drug therapy in the treatment of vestibular migraine is that there has traditionally been a lack of consistently-used criteria for diagnosing vestibular migraine[125]. Consequently, it has been difficult to compare treatment methods given that diagnosis of the disease may differ between practitioners. Hopefully the establishment of vestibular migraine diagnostic criteria in recent years can help improve accuracy of vestibular migraine recognition[55] which can in turn improve the effectiveness of drug therapy. In other words, an individual with migraine and – coincidentally – a disease such as BPPV that may have previously been treated as migraine-associated vertigo can now be treated as two separate conditions. Furthermore, the relative 'newness' of the diagnostic criteria of vestibular migraine has not allowed for adequate studies to determine proper dosing amounts or dosing schedules that may ultimately have beneficial outcomes once proper pharmaceutical dosing and timelines are better established.

Vestibular Rehabilitation

With some disorders of the inner ear, physical rehabilitation can help improve symptoms in certain individuals. This treatment typically involves specific exercises and/or movements that can be beneficial at helping the brain adjust to the information it receives during a vestibule-related attack. Surprisingly, there is very little research specific to the benefit of vestibular rehabilitation in treating vestibular migraine, particularly in comparison to the amount of research into pharmaceutical treatment. Vestibular rehabilitation is designed to target the physical effects of vestibular migraine such as focusing on compensation tactics to counteract deficits or visual dependence training[143]. Specific to vestibular migraine, one study found that exercises including balance and gait work, habituation, and gaze stability had a positive effect on dizziness; however, the treatment took a minimum of nine weeks to improve dizziness[144]. Another study reported marked improvement in dizziness as well as the number of falls after vestibular-related physical therapy[145]. Clearly, more research is needed in this area.

Supplementation and homeopathic therapy

In addition to the treatments we have discussed so far, there is also a classification of treatments that consist of areas such as homeopathic or naturopathic in design. These treatments typically involve natural substances (e.g. minerals, herbs, etc.) that are largely thought to help the body heal itself. And unlike drugs, supplements consist of nutrients already in our diets such as calcium, magnesium, vitamins, or perhaps food items such as garlic. Because many of these treatments are already a part of our diet, one positive aspect of supplements and many homeopathic treatments is that they are largely considered a safe alternative to drug therapy. Whereas pharmaceuticals attempt to alter or stop a physiologic process from occurring, supplements serve to provide ample amounts of a particular substance to our body. Furthermore, most supplement and homeopathic therapy is relatively inexpensive, particularly in comparison to many migraine and vestibular-related drugs.

This classification of treatments, however, is not without criticism. One common complaint of naturopathic or homeopathic medicine is that there is often a lack of scientific evidence to support the effectiveness of such products. Many of the more established and recognized medical websites tend to limit their mention of – or even exclude – homeopathic-based treatments, while at the same time listing out several pharmaceutical options. I have observed this myself in researching this book, as trying to find supplement- or homeopathic-based medical studies published in reputable journals is difficult. Consequently, patients are often left with anecdotal evidence specific to what is reported on message boards and social media to be beneficial for vestibular migraine. The evidence supporting many of these treatments is often lacking; however, it cannot be ignored that evidence *refuting* these treatments is largely lacking as well.

As evidence of the array of homeopathic treatments available, a quick online search using the keywords *homeopathic vestibular migraine* revealed the following recommended treatment options, among others:

- Magnesium
- Riboflavin (Vitamin B2)
- Capsaicin
- Vertigoheel
- Essential oils
- Cannabidiol (CBD) oil
- Bromine
- Iron
- Conium
- Turmeric
- Ginkgo biloba
- Ginger/Ginger root
- Cocculus indicus

Because of a lack of data supporting their use, it is often up to the patient as to whether they should honor the claims made toward homeopathic and supplement use for the treatment of vestibular migraine. Many of these treatments were listed without any indication of how the purported benefits were obtained; in other words, there was no mention of the study design used to test the stated treatment against a placebo. For example, that quick internet search also revealed a claim that a homeopathic treatment worked as effectively as an anti-vertigo drug for reducing vertigo. This is certainly worth investigating, but it must be remembered that several studies have found that the number of vestibular migraine patients benefitting from drug treatment can be a very small fraction of overall patients; therefore, the aforementioned claims that the homeopathic treatment was *as effective as* a drug could easily be interpreted to mean that both treatments were successful in reducing vertigo. However, if there was no real improvement in vertigo, the same claim could also mean that both treatments had no effect. Therefore, depending on the true outcome specific to the change in vertigo, the claim that the homeopathic treatment is as effective as a drug could technically be correct even if it had no effect!

In order to understand how to investigate those situations where there is not a lot of scientific evidence available to back up a claim, let's look at an example of why it's important to dig deeper into reported claims. Cannabidiol (CBD) oil is often touted as beneficial for treating vestibular conditions. But the majority of known benefit from CBD lies in its ability to suppress some forms of nausea[146]. Without question, nausea is certainly a consistent factor in many vestibular-related conditions. So when asking the question *is CBD effective at treating vestibular migraine*, as a patient you have to carefully analyze the response. If the answer you hear back is 'yes', does that mean *all* aspects of vestibular migraine are helped by CBD? If the answer is instead 'it helps a little', then again – which components of vestibular migraine does it help with? If the reply to the question is 'it helps my nausea', then you have a much more specific answer – and one that is backed up by evidence – allowing you to then look for additional treatments that may be beneficial for the migraine and/or vertigo components of vestibular migraine.

As a patient, it is up to you to perform your own investigation into all treatment options whether pharmaceutical or homeopathic in nature. Understand though, that part of the reason I'm focusing on having you do your due diligence with homeopathic treatments is that they are largely unregulated by the government (in the United States). Supplements are largely viewed by the government as being safe until proven unsafe; therefore, claims are not typically investigated until there is a consistent trend of negative issues occurring. Drugs, on the other hand, are much more regulated, and as such have to go through a very specific process in order to gain approval for use. And drugs are viewed by the government as being unsafe until proven safe through a rigorous research and testing protocol than can take ten years or more and generate a wealth of documents touting every possible result and side effect.

When it comes to homeopathic or supplement-based treatment, remember what we discussed earlier – if you are not having success in your current treatment and there is minimal if any harm in trying a homeopathic treatment, it may well be worth it to give that treatment a shot. Just look at the favorable online reports of products like CBD oil or essential oils as an example of a highly-touted vestibular migraine treatment with minimal, if any, claimed side effects. It's highly unlikely that such high numbers of patients are all mistaken; therefore, it may be a product worth investigating for your own benefit. But before taking any product, consult with your physician and spend time researching not only the benefits but also the reported side effects and complications that can occur when using the product.

Conclusion

Almost any patient afflicted with vestibular migraine will quickly ask the question *how do I treat it.* At present, treatment options are limited and of mixed results. Some patients will note a good deal of improvement to pharmaceutical therapy while others will report no effect or in some cases could be deterred from a significant degree of side effects. Along with any treatment, avoidance of known triggers is essential in order to ensure that an attack is deterred. When known treatments turn out to be ineffective, patients often turn to less-reliable and less-proven measures, which may or may not produce results. However, if there is no expected harm to the patient and the treatment does not worsen symptoms, there is typically little reason not to try these alternative options. Based on the limited success of various treatments, much research needs to be done in the area of treating acute vestibular migraine attacks and also preventing future attacks.

Chapter 8: Related Conditions

VESTIBULAR MIGRAINE IS ONE of the most common causes of vertigo[147]. Unfortunately, it also shares symptoms with many other conditions that can cause dizziness, vertigo, unsteadiness, and headache. As we have discussed, this similarity that vestibular migraine shares with several other medical conditions can be a sort of hindrance given that the symptoms of these other conditions can interfere with the diagnosis for vestibular migraine. This chapter serves to outline several of these other conditions in order to highlight the similarities that they share with vestibular migraine. Recognizing the characteristics of each disorder specific to what is similar with – as well as different from – vestibular migraine can help not only differentiate each condition but also put the patient on track for the appropriate treatment.

Ménière's disease

Ménière's disease is an illness thought to result from problems with the fluid regulation system of the inner ear.

Ménière's patients typically experience an ongoing degree of unsteadiness and ear pressure or fullness intermixed with bouts of acute vertigo, nausea, and vomiting that can last several hours or more. Due in large part to the complexity and sensitivity of the vestibular system, Ménière's remains a complicated disease. While the acute vertigo attacks of Ménière's can be extremely debilitating, much like the attacks associated with vestibular migraine, those attacks can be followed by months or years of almost no symptoms.

Several theorized causes of Ménière's have been proposed, including body water regulation issues, endolymph reabsorption anomalies, vascular abnormalities, and autoimmune factors. Of these possible causes, fluid regulation in the middle ear is considered to be one of the main triggers of Ménière's[148]. For example, water channels, which regulate the transport of water across membranes, have been implicated as a possible main cause of Ménière's[149]. This theory results from the idea that unexpected reductions or increases in the number of water channels can influence the balance of fluid on each side of a membrane, and any alteration in fluid balance can have negative consequences in the equilibrium system of the ear.

Similarly, some researchers suggest that Ménière's patients have a diminished capacity to regulate fluid within their inner ear[150]. Consequently, fluctuations in the inner ear fluid are not well tolerated in Ménière's patients. This is thought to lead to fluid imbalances that contribute to many of the symptoms encountered by Ménière's patients. Electrolytes such as sodium that are known to play a role in the body's fluid regulation are commonly restricted in

Ménière's patients in order to reduce potential fluctuations within the middle ear.

Other theorized causes of Ménière's disease include autoimmune disorders[151], the herpes virus[152], cervical (i.e. neck) disorders[153] and stress[154]. Whereas no definitive cause of Ménière's has been discovered, it is vital that research continue to investigate these and all logical possibilities to determine the potential link and/or similarities between Ménière's and vestibular migraine. At present there remains no cure for Ménière's, though symptoms can often be controlled through the aforementioned sodium restriction, medication, intratympanic steroid injection, and if necessary, surgical procedures on the middle ear.

Acoustic Neuroma

Acoustic neuromas, or 'vestibular schwannomas', are slow growing benign tumors[155] of the eighth (vestibulocochlear) nerve[156]. The tumor is slow-growing, but can interfere with other structures of the inner ear[157]. With an incidence of 1 in 100,000, acoustic neuromas are quite rare and mainly affect older adults[157]. The most common symptoms of acoustic neuroma include tinnitus as well as hearing loss in the affected ear[157]. Up to 15% of patients do not experience hearing loss or tinnitus but do report vertigo, and that vertigo often results in them tending to drift to one side.

Because they are rather slow-growing, treatment for an acoustic neuroma can range from conservative methods such as simple long-term observation to the more intensive use of radiation[158] and/or surgical removal[156, 159].

Benign positional paroxysmal vertigo

As we have discussed, one of the most common vertigo conditions seen in primary care is benign positional paroxysmal vertigo (BPPV)[160]. Despite the long name, each word plays a role in describing what occurs with the disease. Most patients with this relatively harmless (benign) condition describe sudden (paroxysmal) bouts of vertigo that occur with certain (positional) head positions.

The mechanism involved in BPPV is thought to be due to the presence of loose crystals (i.e. otoliths) within the semicircular canals of the ear. As otoliths are not normally present within the semicircular canals, certain head movements cause the loose otoliths to contact the delicate hair cells of the semicircular canals, causing them to trigger and falsely indicate body motion when the head is in particular positions. For example, patients with BPPV often report short bouts of vertigo when looking upwards or rolling over in bed[161]. Furthermore, nausea and vomiting can occur with more severe cases such as *intractable BPPV*.

Diagnosis of BPPV typically involves a thorough medical history and evaluation along with manipulating the head in an attempt to reproduce the symptoms. Most commonly, the Dix-Hallpike maneuver is used to attempt to reproduce the symptoms of BPPV. For this procedure, the patient is seated on a table and their head position is manipulated while the patient is put through a series of specific body positions. Because the otoliths will typically induce nystagmus along with vertigo, the patient's eyes are observed for nystagmus along with any patient-reported vertigo. Results of the Dix-Hallpike test are relatively reliable, being able to correctly identify patients with BPPV 83% of the time while correctly excluding patients without BPPV 52% of the time[160].

For those patients testing positive for BPPV, vestibular rehabilitation as well as canalith repositioning (e.g. Epley maneuver) are relatively successful. Vestibular rehabilitation typically consists of a series of head and/or body motions which may involve fixation of the eye on a single point. Pharmaceutical treatments are not recommended for use in the treatment of BPPV as research has shown no benefit[162]. It is also possible that BBPV symptoms return.

Vestibular neuritis

Vestibular neuritis is associated with vertigo, nausea, vomiting, and imbalance, and is thought to be due to viral inflammation of the vestibular nerve[163]. The condition is acute in nature with symptoms lasting from a few days to several weeks, but up to half of those suffering from vestibular neuritis can experience symptoms much longer[164]. Vestibular neuritis has been reported to account for nearly 10% of all dizziness-related medical visits[165]. Interestingly, viral epidemics trigger an increased incidence of vestibular neuritis, lending evidence to its likely inflammatory origins[166].

Patients exhibiting vestibular neuritis will present with acute, severe vertigo[161]. The most severe attacks can last for one to two days and then gradually subside over the following weeks. Motion may worsen the vertigo, and some patients experience nausea and vomiting in conjunction with the vertigo[161]. Additional symptoms often include nystagmus along with a walking pattern in which the patient tends to lean toward the affected ear's side.

Treatment of vestibular neuritis includes symptomatic care along with vestibular rehabilitation, which can begin as soon as tolerable after cessation of immediate symptoms[161]. Vestibular rehabilitation has been reported to be successful when compared against no therapy[167]. If vestibular neuritis is severe, short-term hospitalization may be required[161].

Concussion

It might seem a little odd to include a condition such as concussion in with a chapter about vestibular-related medical conditions, but I think you will see that concussion certainly belongs in a discussion of conditions whose symptoms resemble that of vestibular migraine. Concussion is a type of traumatic brain injury that most often results from a direct hit to the head or a type of injury (e.g. whiplash) that causes the brain to move rapidly within the skull. Concussions are not uncommon, with over 3 million concussions thought to occur per year in the United States[168]. The cause of concussion can vary by age, as children and older adults most commonly experience concussion as a result of falls, while in adults the most common cause is motor vehicle accidents[169]. Athletic participation, especially high-contact sports such as football, hockey, or boxing is also a common cause for concussion and even includes a separate classification as *sport-related concussion*.

Like many vestibular-related symptoms, imaging through x-ray, MRI, CT scan, etc. are rather ineffective at diagnosing concussion. Therefore, diagnosis is typically reliant upon the patient's history, description of the event that caused the concussion, and their symptoms. The range of symptoms that can occur in response to concussion can vary but do have a close resemblance to many of the symptoms of vestibular migraine. Typically, symptoms of concussion are classified into three areas – cognitive, emotional, and psychological. Cognitive symptoms include difficulty concentrating or thinking (i.e. 'brain fog') in addition to difficulty with information retention. Emotional symptoms of concussion can include irritability, sadness, or general nervousness. Physical symptoms probably have the most similarity to vestibular migraine as they can include headache, blurry vision, nausea and/or vomiting, sensitivity to light or noise, and imbalance issues, among others[169]. With such similarity in symptoms between vestibular migraine and concussion, particularly among athletes or those who are susceptible to head-trauma events, it is somewhat easy to understand how vestibular migraine may be misinterpreted as a concussion event.

Treatment of concussion is generally successful at relieving the associated symptoms. One of the first lines of treatment for concussion is rest. This includes both cognitive rest such as avoiding or reducing tasks that require a significant amount of 'thinking' (e.g. homework, computer use, etc.) as well as physical rest that avoids strenuous activity. Avoidance of associated triggers such as bright lights and loud noise is also recommended[170].

One of the positive aspects of concussion is that, unlike vestibular migraines currently, proper treatment generally results in a full recovery. Some individuals do have extended symptoms (e.g. 3 or more months), but the majority of individuals who suffer a concussion have relief of symptoms in a week or less and are typically allowed to resume activity. Having a concussion can predispose an individual to having a future concussion, so care must be taken to limit the opportunity for future concussions to occur.

Conclusion

It has been mentioned several times in this book that vestibular migraine often presents similar to other medical conditions. This chapter was designed to outline several of those conditions so as to highlight the similarities and make you as a patient aware of the most common symptoms. Some conditions such as vestibular migraine and Ménière's may appear with little warning, while others such as concussion typically involve some sort of head trauma. However, many of the conditions discussed in this chapter can also arise after head trauma, thereby complicating the diagnosis. In many cases, the key to separating one medical condition from the rest is to outline a clear medical history specific to symptoms, duration, severity, and when the symptoms started, then apply the proper diagnostic criteria to each. Therefore, as a patient it is important to provide precise detail to your physician in order to assist them in making a proper diagnosis. It is equally important as a patient to ensure that you provide updates to your physician specific to the symptoms you experience as well as your response to treatment.

Chapter 9: Quality of Life

THE TERM "QUALITY OF LIFE" represents the degree to which an individual is able to maintain an acceptable degree of health, comfort, and happiness in their life. In medicine, as a condition worsens or as it negatively impacts their daily life more, quality of life tends to decrease. There is little doubt that vestibular migraine has a significant impact on an individual's quality of life, particularly the degree to which a patient has vestibular migraine as well as the frequency of attacks.

As with treatment, outlining quality of life for a vestibular migraine sufferer can be somewhat difficult because there are multiple components to evaluate. For example, the headache that a sufferer experiences may not be problematic, but the random attacks of vertigo might be. In such cases it might be more relevant to document the impact of vertigo on quality of life rather than documenting 'vestibular migraine' itself. Yet as we have shown, vestibular migraine can carry with it a separate set of negative influences. For example, almost half of individuals attending a 'dizziness clinic' in Germany or China report anxiety and depression[171, 172]. While either condition can be problematic on its own, vestibular migraine still adds another component to deal with. These aspects can outline some of the difficulty that lies in establishing quality of life specifically for vestibular migraine; therefore, it can also be relevant to look at quality of life values for migraine as well as for vertigo separately, along with quality of life for other vestibular conditions such as Ménière's or BPPV.

Research has shown that both vestibular migraine and migraine patients have more anxiety and apprehension than healthy individuals[94]. Furthermore, these patients displayed both more panic symptoms and more illness phobias than healthy people. Among migraine and vestibular migraine patients, vestibular migraine sufferers were more anxious and more worried about not being able to find easy 'escape routes' when in public (i.e. agoraphobia). Similarly, vestibular migraine patients, along with Meniere's disease sufferers, exhibit more frequent anxiety and depression than patients with vestibular neuritis or BPPV[172].

As to quality of life specific to vestibular migraine, the research is lacking. One study from 2006 did show that health-related quality of life is lower than among non-dizzy individuals, but the authors of that study pointed out that there were a low number of vestibular migraine patients, which may have influenced the study results[67]. However, the same authors outlined how vestibular migraine can disrupt daily life. For example, 40% of vestibular migraine patients had to take sick leave from work. Separately, almost 40% of participants in the study had used medication for their vertigo, but only one-third of those individuals reported a favorable response to the medication. And it was also interesting to learn how patients in the study self-reported the impact of vestibular migraine on their life. About 21% claimed that their vestibular migraine was 'mild'. Another 46% reported it as 'moderate', and 33% as 'severe'. Severe was described in the study as 'daily activities had to be abandoned'. Therefore, according to at least one study, approximately 33% of people with vestibular migraine cannot perform their normal daily activities when experiencing a vestibular migraine attack. Clearly, there is a significant impact on an individual's quality of life with vestibular migraine, even for moderately-affected individuals who report 'interference with daily activities'.

Personal stories

Despite a relative lack of scientific data specific to vestibular migraine's reported quality of life, I thought that there's probably no better way to capture the everyday impact of vestibular migraine than to hear from patients who are living with the disease. Therefore, I asked several patients to answer one question: "what is it like to live with vestibular migraine on a daily basis?". I leave you with their answers to close out this chapter. But use caution in reading the next few pages, as some responses are far from favorable and make no attempt to cast vestibular migraine in any kind of a positive light. Still, I think that allowing patients to state what they truly feel about living with this disease is the best way to capture the effect and impact that vestibular migraine can have on an individual's quality of life.

- *My average day with VM consists of me being dizzy, feeling drunk, and hungover at the same time. I have constant head and eye pressure. My head is pounding. I feel off-balance. My neck hurts and feels heavy. This is all 24/7. I can no longer drive. I now have crippling anxiety and depression. I have pondered taking my life on more than one occasion. I feel worthless, and feel as if I have no value as a member of society, as a wife, as a mother, as a grandma. I have lost my independence. I have aged so much since this began. I look 20 years older. I mainly just "get through the day". I wish people could understand how much I suffer. There are not words to describe it. To most I appear normal. My family definitely sees the change, and what this has done to me. However they will never understand – how could they? This is invisible for the most part. I wish doctors would stop saying it's "just anxiety", and telling me I need mental help. I am sick of trying drugs that often make me worse. This is becoming an epidemic, with so many people affected. We need a cure! We need help, patience, understanding, and doctors who care and don't give up on us.*

- *When you have VM you never know how you are going to feel day by day. I have to monitor what I do constantly. Something as simple as turning my head too quickly can send me into an "episode" causing me to be off-balance for several hours. It is next to impossible to make plans because I don't know if I'll have to cancel or worse, go and suffer the consequences. On vacations, skull crushing migraines can leave me trapped in a hotel room for days while everyone else has fun. I have been in work meetings when my brain and my mouth don't cooperate with each other. My coworkers just stare at me when this happens. Sometimes at work I will just refuse to speak and I'm sure my bosses just think I'm being difficult. Public speaking of any kind is out of the question as I will pass out. Financially, even with insurance VM can be draining. Copays for neurologists, PCP, cardiologists and ENTs add up quickly. My prescriptions easily cost hundreds of dollars each month. I have frequently only filled partial prescriptions because of financial reasons. Because I have symptoms most every day, VM can be very depressing and isolating. I have had terrible migraines for 19 years and was just recently diagnosed with VM.*

- *The worst thing, besides being dizzy and disoriented, is when my husband doesn't understand why I can't complete a sentence or say the wrong word when I mean something else! I feel like he's picking on me and usually I end up crying and going to bed!*

- *I used to refer it as "my Ozzy Osbourne syndrome" because not long after mine started to be bad his reality show was on. Remember how he'd shuffle and mumble? That's how I felt during an episode.*

- *Having VM is like having a part time job. I have so many things that I must do to try and ward off my so called silent headaches. Shopping and cooking are now more time consuming, as I try to follow the 'Heal Your*

Headache' diet. I have a visual therapy and a physiotherapy appointment every week. I have eye exercises that I must do every day. I also exercise every day for an hour, as this is an important factor in trying to stop my symptoms. I sometimes also do balance exercises. And most important of all I spend time every day trying to educate myself on this illness. I am describing a good day. On a bad day, I can't do anything. If I was not retired, I could not fight this illness as effectively as I have.

- *In the first 5 minutes of the movie Adrift, a woman wakes up on a sinking, rocking ship with a nasty head injury. This is what life with VM can feel like 24 hours a day, 7 days a week, for months or years on end.*

- *VM is not just a simple headache where you take a pill and you are better. VM is more like someone has stomped on your brain, and you have a concussion. The side effects are many, and you never know when you are going to have a bad day. I want people to know it is like having a brain injury. For me the drunk dizzy feeling never goes away. I want to spin people around in an office chair, and then say, this is how I feel most of the time.*

- *Symptoms begin with classical migraines, usually a change in attitude, like being really short tempered. Vision becomes distorted, sometimes blacked out on one side, sometimes stars, and things become disoriented, things seem far and then close. Around 3 to 10 minutes after, the nystagmus hits, sometimes accompanied by headaches, sometimes not. Chest pains are almost always with it, and the mouth starts to taste metallic. Nausea hits shortly thereafter. The vertigo is violent, much worse than that from Ménière's and doesn't let up. On occasion the body is in so much pain, moving a toe makes it feel like my head is going to crack open.*

During an attack, if it wasn't for my family, I'd wish I was dead. Sounds over-dramatic, but this really is how it feels. It is agony.

Conclusion

THROUGHOUT THIS BOOK we have outlined the effects of the frustrating, often debilitating condition of vestibular migraine. Despite being one of the most common diseases for causing dizziness, vestibular migraine has only in the past couple of decades began to gain traction in the medical world. The intent of this book was to bring you some clarity into the suspected causes as well as treatment options available for vestibular migraine. And hopefully, you can use the information you learned and improve some aspect of your life with vestibular migraine.

I have written several patient-oriented books on topics relating to the labyrinth system of the ear. Without a doubt, this book has been the most difficult of them all to write. The complexities of vestibular migraine relating to how little we know about it just don't provide a good template by which to organize the available information into a structured set of chapters. For example, we discussed how most of the treatment for vestibular migraine is based on protocols used for migraine. Yet, migraine itself is largely related to headache and often has no vertigo component. In modeling treatments after migraine alone, patients with vestibular migraine have a significant aspect of their disease (i.e. vestibular-based factors) left unaccounted for. This in turn made the research for this book quite difficult at times in trying to separate the available literature specific to migraine from that of vestibular migraine (and also migraine-related vertigo!). I often had to read and then re-read the studies to ensure that I was not mixing up the migraine causes or treatment with that suspected of vestibular migraine. That's one of the many reasons I take pride in providing you the reader a bibliography that lists every resource I used in this book, so that you can perform your own research and learn more along the way.

But quite honestly, I also am certain that the frustration I felt in researching this book pales immensely to what vestibular migraine patients themselves often experience on a daily basis.

One of the most disheartening things I learned in writing this book is that there just isn't much encouraging news out there about promising treatments or likely cures. On the one hand, I as a Ménière's patient have tempered my outlook for expecting good news in the area of vestibular research, given that many related conditions have a similar bleak outlook. But then there's also vestibular conditions like BPPV which can often be fixed in one office visit. And listening to the stories of patients living with vestibular migraine every day, I can't help but wonder what they rely on for daily motivation.

For patients, the poor outlook combined with the sometimes-incapacitating effects of vestibular migraine can often lead to desperate measures. And desperation can lead to a willingness to try anything to stop the dizziness, vertigo, and often constant anxiety. As a patient, you must remain vigilant in what you are willing to try in terms of treatments in order to get some degree of relief. Many people are out to make a quick buck, and desperation can have a magnetic effect on these people. Beware of 'cures' as well as treatments that just seem too good to be true, particularly if there is a significant financial cost tied to trying the treatment. Instead, work with your physician to develop a tailored and structured treatment plan that best fits *you*, and maintain a strong communication line with your physician in order to provide him or her valuable updates as to your successes or regressions.

Along these lines, I will be the first to say that it can be frustrating to watch the pace of progress in the area of vestibular treatments. However, it is important for you to understand that medicine and research are always going on behind the scenes to find a cure. It may not appear that way, or it may not be happening fast enough, but progress is being pursued. A vestibular physician once told me "*We have egos. We _want_ to be the one to find a cure*". What this person was describing is the drive and competitiveness that researchers have towards being the one who discovers 'the' cure for a condition. The cure that will get their name assigned to the treatment, much like Dr. Epley and his success at treating traditional BPPV. The cure that will bring complete relief to literally millions of people. The process in developing this cure, though, requires often years-long studies, approvals, grants, and patient compliance, and it is not a straight path but rather a winding, convoluted trip from start to finish. And given vestibular migraine's relatively short history, the disorder has a lot of catching up to do in order to match what we know about longer-studied areas such as Ménière's and tinnitus.

I hope that this book has brought you 'something' in return for the time you have spent reading it. That something may be an answer you have been seeking, or a better understanding of your condition or perhaps even a topic to bring up with your physician at your next appointment. What I don't want this book to do is to detract from your hope or your drive to push through each day while waiting for improvement. I set out to write each of my books with the intent of providing information to the reader; I am not selling them anything, directing them to my website for more information, or injecting bias such as might occur if I only tell them the 'good news' about their condition. Rather, I want to provide information to them, written in a way that hopefully they understand, with the goal of empowering them as a patient. There is a purported Native American proverb that states *Tell me and I'll forget; Show me, and I may not remember; Involve me, and I'll understand.* My intent for this book was to involve you in the process of discovery in order to help you understand the complexity of this miserable disease. So, as I discovered something of relevance in my research, I included it in the book so that you can better understand the complexity of this disease. The end result is that I hope you are able to walk away from this book with a better understanding of your condition. I certainly know that I have personally gained a tremendous understanding about vestibular migraine.

In closing, I wholeheartedly wish you the best of luck on your journey with vestibular migraine.

Glossary

Acoustic neuroma: a benign tumor that grows on one of the nerves associated with the ear

Ampulla: A bulbous area near the end of the semicircular canal that contains the cupula

Anxiety: any of a group of psychiatric disorders that leads to a feeling of extreme fear, panic, and worry

Aura: a sensation indicative of a warning that precedes a migraine

Benign: not harmful

Benign paroxysmal positional vertigo: a condition of the inner ear thought to result from loose otoliths that can cause severe bouts of vertigo in response to certain head positions

Confounder: a factor in an experiment that can influence the results and must be accounted for

Control group: In experimental design, the group that does not receive the experimental condition but is otherwise treated identical to the experimental group

Cupula: A structure at the end of each semicircular canal that detects fluid motion within the canals during head movement

Definite risk factor: a component directly responsible for causing a condition or symptom

Dizziness: a sensation that results in the patient feeling as if he or she is spinning or moving while remaining stationary

Endolymph: the potassium-rich fluid contained within the membranous labyrinth of the ear

Equilibrium: a state of overall balance

Experimental group: In experimental design, the group that receives the experimental condition but is otherwise treated identical to the control group

Hair Cell: sensory receptors located within the auditory and vestibular organs of the ear that transmit a signal to the brain in response to detection of head movement or sound vibrations

Hypothesis: a prediction made based on available evidence

Indefinite risk factor: a component that may play a role in developing or worsening a condition or symptom

Inner Ear: the portion of the ear within the temporal bone that contains the semicircular canals and cochlea

Labyrinth: the portion of the ear containing the hearing and balance organs

Ménière's Disease: a condition of the inner ear comprised of symptoms that include vertigo, tinnitus, hearing loss, and the sensation of ear fullness

Middle Ear: the central cavity of the inner ear comprised of the empty space within the temporal bone located inside of the eardrum

Migraine: a complex neurological disease causing a headache of varying intensity, often accompanied by nausea and sensitivity to light and sound

Nystagmus: involuntary eye movement

Oscillopsia: a visual condition in which the patient reports that objects in their field of view appear to move in circles or rapid motions

Otolith: a small crystalline structure of the inner ear that plays a role in balance and equilibrium

Outer Ear: That portion of the ear that is visible, along with the auditory canal

Phonophobia: a sensitivity to sound

Photophobia: a sensitivity to light

Pinna: the external portion of the ear

Quality of Life: a person's perceived ability to enjoy normal activities

Receptor: a small structure in the body that responds to a chemical message within the body

Saccule: a structure within the vestibular responsible for providing feedback about vertical head motion

Secondary tinnitus: tinnitus that occurs in response to a recognized medical condition

Semicircular canals: Three passages within the temporal bone responsible for providing feedback regarding rotational head movement

Subjective tinnitus: tinnitus that is only detectable by the patient

Symptom: a physical or mental aspect of a medical condition that is typically evident only to the patient

Temporal bone: A bone that is positioned at the side and base of the skull which houses the vestibular and hearing organs

Utricle: A structure within the vestibule responsible for providing feedback about horizontal head motion

Vertigo: a sensation of spinning that is usually accompanied by a sudden loss of balance

Vertigo – external: a type of vertigo in which the external environment seems to be moving in relation to the body

Vertigo – internal: a type of vertigo in which the body feels as though it is moving in response to or 'through' the environment

Vestibular nerve: the eighth cranial nerve, responsible for transmitting hearing and sensory information from the inner ear to the brain.

Vestibule: a sensory-based organ within the inner ear that is responsible for helping the body maintain postural equilibrium

References

1. Stolte, B., et al., *Vestibular migraine*. Cephalalgia, 2015. **35**(3): p. 262-270.
2. Ekdale, E.G., *Form and function of the mammalian inner ear*. Journal of anatomy, 2016. **228**(2): p. 324-337.
3. Murayama, E., et al., *Otolith matrix proteins OMP-1 and Otolin-1 are necessary for normal otolith growth and their correct anchoring onto the sensory maculae*. Mechanisms of development, 2005. **122**(6): p. 791-803.
4. Walther, L.E., et al., *Detection of human utricular otoconia degeneration in vital specimen and implications for benign paroxysmal positional vertigo*. European Archives of Oto-Rhino-Laryngology, 2014. **271**(12): p. 3133-3138.
5. Andrade, L.R., et al., *Immunogold TEM of otoconin 90 and otolin–relevance to mineralization of otoconia, and pathogenesis of benign positional vertigo*. Hearing research, 2012. **292**(1-2): p. 14-25.
6. Parham, K., *Benign paroxysmal positional vertigo: an integrated perspective*. Advances in otolaryngology, 2014. **2014**.
7. Giacomini, P.G., et al., *Recurrent paroxysmal positional vertigo related to oral contraceptive treatment*. Gynecological endocrinology, 2006. **22**(1): p. 5-8.
8. Schuknecht, H. and R. Ruby, *Cupulolithiasis*, in *Otophysiology*. 1973, Karger Publishers. p. 434-443.
9. Pérez-Vázquez, P. and V. Franco-Gutiérrez, *Treatment of benign paroxysmal positional vertigo. A clinical review.* 收藏, 2017. **4**: p. 002.

10. Lawal, O. and D. Navaratnam, *Causes of Central Vertigo*, in *Diagnosis and Treatment of Vestibular Disorders*. 2019, Springer. p. 363-375.
11. Peng, B., *Cervical vertigo: historical reviews and advances*. World neurosurgery, 2018. **109**: p. 347-350.
12. Labuguen, R.H., *Initial evaluation of vertigo*. Am Fam Physician, 2006. **73**(2): p. 244-51.
13. Lee, A., *Diagnosing the cause of vertigo: a practical approach*. Hong Kong Med J, 2012. **18**(4): p. 327-32.
14. Glover, J.C., *Vestibular System*, in *Encyclopedia of Neuroscience*, L.R. Squire, Editor. 2004, Academic Press: Oxford. p. 127-132.
15. American Migraine Foundation. *What is Migraine*. Available from: https://americanmigrainefoundation.org/resource-library/what-is-migraine/.
16. Stewart, W.F., A. Shechter, and B.K. Rasmussen, *Migraine prevalence. A review of population-based studies*. Neurology, 1994. **44**(6 Suppl 4): p. S17-23.
17. Woldeamanuel, Y.W. and R.P. Cowan, *Migraine affects 1 in 10 people worldwide featuring recent rise: a systematic review and meta-analysis of community-based studies involving 6 million participants*. Journal of the Neurological Sciences, 2017. **372**: p. 307-315.
18. Lipton, R.B., et al., *Prevalence and burden of migraine in the United States: data from the American Migraine Study II*. Headache: The Journal of Head and Face Pain, 2001. **41**(7): p. 646-657.
19. Leonardi, M., et al., *The global burden of migraine: measuring disability in headache disorders with WHO's*

Classification of Functioning, Disability and Health (ICF). The journal of headache and pain, 2005. **6**(6): p. 429.

20. Radtke, A., et al., *Migraine and Ménière's disease: is there a link?* Neurology, 2002. **59**(11): p. 1700-1704.
21. Ferrari, M.D., et al., *Migraine pathophysiology: lessons from mouse models and human genetics.* The Lancet Neurology, 2015. **14**(1): p. 65-80.
22. Lewis, D.W., *Pediatric migraine.* Neurologic clinics, 2009. **27**(2): p. 481-501.
23. Burstein, R., R. Noseda, and D. Borsook, *Migraine: multiple processes, complex pathophysiology.* Journal of Neuroscience, 2015. **35**(17): p. 6619-6629.
24. Goadsby, P.J., et al., *Pathophysiology of migraine: a disorder of sensory processing.* Physiological reviews, 2017. **97**(2): p. 553-622.
25. Schulte, L.H., T.P. Jürgens, and A. May, *Photo-, osmo-and phonophobia in the premonitory phase of migraine: mistaking symptoms for triggers?* The journal of headache and pain, 2015. **16**(1): p. 14.
26. Dahlem, M.A., et al., *Understanding migraine using dynamic network biomarkers.* Cephalalgia, 2015. **35**(7): p. 627-630.
27. Charles, A.C. and S.M. Baca, *Cortical spreading depression and migraine.* Nature Reviews Neurology, 2013. **9**(11): p. 637.
28. Charles, A. and K. Brennan, *Cortical spreading depression—new insights and persistent questions.* Cephalalgia, 2009. **29**(10): p. 1115-1124.
29. Zhang, X., et al., *Ezogabine (KCNQ2/3 channel opener) prevents delayed activation of meningeal nociceptors if given*

before but not after the occurrence of cortical spreading depression. Epilepsy & Behavior, 2013. **28**(2): p. 243-248.

30. Moskowitz, M. and R. Macfarlane, *Neurovascular and molecular mechanisms in migraine headaches.* Cerebrovascular and brain metabolism reviews, 1993. **5**(3): p. 159-177.

31. Freilinger, T., et al., *Genome-wide association analysis identifies susceptibility loci for migraine without aura.* Nature genetics, 2012. **44**(7): p. 777.

32. Maleki, N., et al., *Concurrent functional and structural cortical alterations in migraine.* Cephalalgia, 2012. **32**(8): p. 607-620.

33. Vos, T., et al., *Global, regional, and national incidence, prevalence, and years lived with disability for 310 diseases and injuries, 1990–2015: a systematic analysis for the Global Burden of Disease Study 2015.* The Lancet, 2016. **388**(10053): p. 1545-1602.

34. Vetvik, K.G. and E.A. MacGregor, *Sex differences in the epidemiology, clinical features, and pathophysiology of migraine.* The Lancet Neurology, 2017. **16**(1): p. 76-87.

35. Rasmussen, B.K. and J. Olesen, *Migraine with aura and migraine without aura: an epidemiological study.* Cephalalgia, 1992. **12**(4): p. 221-228.

36. Kelman, L., *The premonitory symptoms (prodrome): a tertiary care study of 893 migraineurs.* Headache: The Journal of Head and Face Pain, 2004. **44**(9): p. 865-872.

37. Society, H.C.C.o.t.I.H., *The international classification of headache disorders, (beta version).* Cephalalgia, 2013. **33**(9): p. 629-808.

38. Kelman, L. and D. Tanis, *The relationship between migraine pain and other associated symptoms.* Cephalalgia, 2006. **26**(5): p. 548-553.

39. Messali, A., et al., *Direct and indirect costs of chronic and episodic migraine in the United States: A web-based survey.* Headache: The Journal of Head and Face Pain, 2016. **56**(2): p. 306-322.

40. Hu, X.H., et al., *Burden of migraine in the United States: disability and economic costs.* Archives of internal medicine, 1999. **159**(8): p. 813-818.

41. Murray, C.J., et al., *Disability-adjusted life years (DALYs) for 291 diseases and injuries in 21 regions, 1990–2010: a systematic analysis for the Global Burden of Disease Study 2010.* The lancet, 2012. **380**(9859): p. 2197-2223.

42. Vos, T., et al., *Years lived with disability (YLDs) for 1160 sequelae of 289 diseases and injuries 1990–2010: a systematic analysis for the Global Burden of Disease Study 2010.* The lancet, 2012. **380**(9859): p. 2163-2196.

43. Scher, A., et al., *Factors associated with the onset and remission of chronic daily headache in a population-based study.* Pain, 2003. **106**(1-2): p. 81-89.

44. Katsarava, Z., et al., *Incidence and predictors for chronicity of headache in patients with episodic migraine.* Neurology, 2004. **62**(5): p. 788-790.

45. Mathew, N.T., R. Kurman, and F. Perez, *Drug induced refractory headache-clinical features and management.* Headache: The Journal of Head and Face Pain, 1990. **30**(10): p. 634-638.

46. Peterlin, B.L., et al., *Obesity and migraine: the effect of age, gender and adipose tissue distribution.* Headache: The Journal of Head and Face Pain, 2010. **50**(1): p. 52-62.

47.   Bigal, M.E., J.N. Liberman, and R.B. Lipton, *Obesity and migraine: a population study.* Neurology, 2006. **66**(4): p. 545-550.

48.   Ashina, S., et al., *Depression and risk of transformation of episodic to chronic migraine.* The journal of headache and pain, 2012. **13**(8): p. 615.

49.   May, A. and L.H. Schulte, *Chronic migraine: risk factors, mechanisms and treatment.* Nature Reviews Neurology, 2016. **12**(8): p. 455.

50.   Russo, A.F., *Calcitonin gene-related peptide (CGRP): a new target for migraine.* Annual review of pharmacology and toxicology, 2015. **55**: p. 533-552.

51.   Evers, S. and R. Jensen, *Treatment of medication overuse headache–guideline of the EFNS headache panel.* European journal of neurology, 2011. **18**(9): p. 1115-1121.

52.   Lipton, R.B. and S.H. Pearlman, *Transcranial magnetic simulation in the treatment of migraine.* Neurotherapeutics, 2010. **7**(2): p. 204-212.

53.   Powers, S.W., et al., *Cognitive behavioral therapy plus amitriptyline for chronic migraine in children and adolescents: a randomized clinical trial.* Jama, 2013. **310**(24): p. 2622-2630.

54.   Fuller-Thomson, E., M. Schrumm, and S. Brennenstuhl, *Migraine and despair: factors associated with depression and suicidal ideation among Canadian migraineurs in a population-based study.* Depression research and treatment, 2013. **2013**.

55.   Lempert, T., et al., *Vestibular migraine: diagnostic criteria.* Journal of Vestibular Research, 2012. **22**(4): p. 167-172.

56.   Brandt, T. and M. Strupp, *Migraine and vertigo: classification, clinical features, and special treatment considerations.* Headache Currents, 2006. **3**(1): p. 12-19.

57.   Bickerstaff, E., *Impairment of consciousness in migraine.* The Lancet, 1961. **278**(7211): p. 1057-1059.

58.   Lieving, E., *On megrim, sick-headache and some allied disorders.* London: Churchill, 1873.

59.   Kayan, A. and J.D. Hood, *Neuro-otological manifestations of migraine.* Brain, 1984. **107**(4): p. 1123-1142.

60.   Luzeiro, I., et al., *Vestibular migraine: clinical challenges and opportunities for multidisciplinarity.* Behavioural neurology, 2016. **2016**.

61.   Neuhauser, H., et al., *The interrelations of migraine, vertigo, and migrainous vertigo.* Neurology, 2001. **56**(4): p. 436-441.

62.   Millen, S.J., C.M. Schnurr, and B.B. Schnurr, *Vestibular migraine: perspectives of otology versus neurology.* Otology & Neurotology, 2011. **32**(2): p. 330-337.

63.   Mergl, R., et al., *Depressive, anxiety, and somatoform disorders in primary care: prevalence and recognition.* Depression and anxiety, 2007. **24**(3): p. 185-195.

64.   Jensen, R. and L.J. Stovner, *Epidemiology and comorbidity of headache.* The Lancet Neurology, 2008. **7**(4): p. 354-361.

65.   Neuhauser, H., et al., *Epidemiology of vestibular vertigo: a neurotologic survey of the general population.* Neurology, 2005. **65**(6): p. 898-904.

66.   Lempert, T. and H. Neuhauser, *Epidemiology of vertigo, migraine and vestibular migraine.* Journal of neurology, 2009. **256**(3): p. 333-338.

67.   Neuhauser, H., et al., *Migrainous vertigo: prevalence and impact on quality of life.* Neurology, 2006. **67**(6): p. 1028-1033.

68.   Geser, R. and D. Straumann, *Referral and final diagnoses of patients assessed in an academic vertigo center.* Frontiers in neurology, 2012. **3**: p. 169.

69.   Lauritsen, C.G. and M.J. Marmura, *Current treatment options: vestibular migraine.* Current treatment options in neurology, 2017. **19**(11): p. 38.

70.   Dieterich, M. and T. Brandt, *Episodic vertigo related to migraine (90 cases): vestibular migraine?* Journal of neurology, 1999. **246**(10): p. 883-892.

71.   Cass, S.P., et al., *Migraine-related vestibulopathy.* Annals of Otology, Rhinology & Laryngology, 1997. **106**(3): p. 182-189.

72.   Krams, B., et al., *Benign paroxysmal vertigo of childhood: long-term outcome.* Cephalalgia, 2011. **31**(4): p. 439-443.

73.   Oh, A.K., et al., *Familial benign recurrent vertigo.* American journal of medical genetics, 2001. **100**(4): p. 287-291.

74.   Park, J. and E. Viirre, *Vestibular migraine may be an important cause of dizziness/vertigo in perimenopausal period.* Medical hypotheses, 2010. **75**(5): p. 409-414.

75.   Lance, J.W., *Observations on 500 cases of migraine and allied vascular headache.* J Neurol Neurosurg Psychiatry, 2012. **83**(7): p. 673-674.

76.   Sohn, J.-H., *Recent advances in the understanding of vestibular migraine.* Behavioural neurology, 2016. **2016**.

77.   Lempert, T. *Vestibular migraine.* in *Seminars in neurology.* 2013. Thieme Medical Publishers.

78. Furman, J.M., D.A. Marcus, and C.D. Balaban, *Vestibular migraine: clinical aspects and pathophysiology.* The Lancet Neurology, 2013. **12**(7): p. 706-715.

79. Calhoun, A.H., et al., *The point prevalence of dizziness or vertigo in migraine–and factors that influence presentation.* Headache: The Journal of Head and Face Pain, 2011. **51**(9): p. 1388-1392.

80. Vass, Z., et al., *Direct evidence of trigeminal innervation of the cochlear blood vessels.* Neuroscience, 1998. **84**(2): p. 559-567.

81. Marano, E., et al., *Trigeminal stimulation elicits a peripheral vestibular imbalance in migraine patients.* Headache: the Journal of Head and Face Pain, 2005. **45**(4): p. 325-331.

82. Radtke, A., et al., *Vestibular migraine: long-term follow-up of clinical symptoms and vestibulo-cochlear findings.* Neurology, 2012. **79**(15): p. 1607-1614.

83. Murdin, L., P. Premachandra, and R. Davies, *Sensory dysmodulation in vestibular migraine: an otoacoustic emission suppression study.* The Laryngoscope, 2010. **120**(8): p. 1632-1636.

84. Lewis, R.F., et al., *Dynamic tilt thresholds are reduced in vestibular migraine.* Journal of Vestibular Research, 2011. **21**(6): p. 323-330.

85. Goadsby, P.J., R.B. Lipton, and M.D. Ferrari, *Migraine — current understanding and treatment.* New England journal of medicine, 2002. **346**(4): p. 257-270.

86. Russo, A., et al., *Abnormal thalamic function in patients with vestibular migraine.* Neurology, 2014. **82**(23): p. 2120-2126.

87. Messina, R., et al., *Structural brain abnormalities in patients with vestibular migraine.* Journal of neurology, 2017. **264**(2): p. 295-303.

88. Von Brevern, M. and T. Lempert, *Vestibular migraine,* in *Handbook of clinical neurology.* 2016, Elsevier. p. 301-316.

89. Goto, F., T. Tsutsumi, and K. Ogawa, *The clinical features of migraine-associated vertigo.* Nihon Jibiinkoka Gakkai Kaiho, 2013. **116**(8): p. 953-959.

90. Qiu, F., et al., *An analysis of clinical features of 226 vestibular migraine patients.* Zhonghua nei ke za zhi, 2014. **53**(12): p. 961-963.

91. Johnson, G.D., *Medical management of migraine-related dizziness and vertigo.* The Laryngoscope, 1998. **108**(S85): p. 1-28.

92. Colombo, B., *Migraine: pathophysiology and classification,* in *Vestibular migraine and related syndromes.* 2014, Springer. p. 1-17.

93. Lempert, T., H. Neuhauser, and R.B. Daroff, *Vertigo as a symptom of migraine.* Annals of the New York Academy of Sciences, 2009. **1164**(1): p. 242-251.

94. Kutay, Ö., et al., *Vestibular migraine patients are more anxious than migraine patients without vestibular symptoms.* Journal of neurology, 2017. **264**(1): p. 37-41.

95. Brandt, T., *Vertigo: its multisensory syndromes.* 2013: Springer Science & Business Media.

96. von Brevern, M., et al., *Migrainous vertigo presenting as episodic positional vertigo.* Neurology, 2004. **62**(3): p. 469-472.

97. Martinez, E., et al., *Clinical characteristics of vestibular migraine: considerations in a series of 41 patients.* Revista de neurologia, 2017. **64**(1): p. 1-6.

98.   Waterston, J., *Chronic migrainous vertigo.* Journal of Clinical Neuroscience, 2004. **11**(4): p. 384-388.
99.   Vuković, V., et al., *Prevalence of vertigo, dizziness, and migrainous vertigo in patients with migraine.* Headache: The Journal of Head and Face Pain, 2007. **47**(10): p. 1427-1435.
100.   Neuhauser, H., et al. *Population-based epidemiological evidence for the link between dizziness and migraine.* in *25th Barany Society Meeting, Kyoto:* p. 2008.
101.   Hilton, D.B. and C. Shermetaro, *Headache, Migraine-Associated Vertigo (Vestibular Migraine),* in *StatPearls [Internet].* 2018, StatPearls Publishing.
102.   Furman, J.M. and C.D. Balaban, *Vestibular migraine.* Annals of the New York Academy of Sciences, 2015. **1343**(1): p. 90-96.
103.   Furman, J., et al., *Migraine–anxiety related dizziness (MARD): a new disorder?* 2005, BMJ Publishing Group Ltd.
104.   Van Ombergen, A., et al., *Vestibular migraine in an otolaryngology clinic: prevalence, associated symptoms, and prophylactic medication effectiveness.* Otology & Neurotology, 2015. **36**(1): p. 133-138.
105.   McKeown, R.E., et al., *The impact of case definition on attention-deficit/hyperactivity disorder prevalence estimates in community-based samples of school-aged children.* Journal of the American Academy of Child & Adolescent Psychiatry, 2015. **54**(1): p. 53-61.
106.   Radtke, A., et al., *Vestibular migraine–validity of clinical diagnostic criteria.* Cephalalgia, 2011. **31**(8): p. 906-913.

107. Langhagen, T., et al., *Vestibular migraine in children and adolescents: clinical findings and laboratory tests.* Frontiers in neurology, 2015. **5**: p. 292.

108. Society, H.C.C.o.t.I.H., *Classification and diagnostic criteria for headache disorders, cranial neuralgias and facial pain.* Cephalalgia, 1988. **8**(7): p. 1-96.

109. Olesen, J. and T. Steiner, *The International classification of headache disorders, 2nd edn (ICDH-II).* 2004, BMJ Publishing Group Ltd.

110. Li, C.-M., et al., *Epidemiology of dizziness and balance problems in children in the United States: a population-based study.* The Journal of pediatrics, 2016. **171**: p. 240-247. e3.

111. Brodsky, J.R., B.A. Cusick, and G. Zhou, *Evaluation and management of vestibular migraine in children: experience from a pediatric vestibular clinic.* European Journal of Paediatric Neurology, 2016. **20**(1): p. 85-92.

112. Lee, J.D., et al., *Prevalence of vestibular and balance disorders in children and adolescents according to age: a multi-center study.* International journal of pediatric otorhinolaryngology, 2017. **94**: p. 36-39.

113. Balatsouras, D.G., et al., *Etiology of vertigo in children.* International journal of pediatric otorhinolaryngology, 2007. **71**(3): p. 487-494.

114. Jahn, K., et al., *Vertigo and dizziness in childhood– update on diagnosis and treatment.* Neuropediatrics, 2011. **42**(04): p. 129-134.

115. Gruber, M., et al., *Vertigo in children and adolescents: characteristics and outcome.* The Scientific World Journal, 2012. **2012**.

116. Humphriss, R.L. and A.J. Hall, *Dizziness in 10 year old children: an epidemiological study.* International journal of pediatric otorhinolaryngology, 2011. **75**(3): p. 395-400.

117. Bárány Society. *About the Bárány Society.* 2019; Available from: http://baranysociety.nl/home%20page/aboutbarany/index.html.

118. Brantberg, K. and R.W. Baloh, *Similarity of vertigo attacks due to Meniere's disease and benign recurrent vertigo, both with and without migraine.* Acta oto-laryngologica, 2011. **131**(7): p. 722-727.

119. Ishiyama, A., K.M. Jacobson, and R.W. Baloh, *Migraine and benign positional vertigo.* Annals of Otology, Rhinology & Laryngology, 2000. **109**(4): p. 377-380.

120. Colombo, B. and R. Teggi, *Vestibular migraine: who is the patient?* Neurological Sciences, 2017. **38**(1): p. 107-110.

121. Lee, S.-H. and J.S. Kim, *Benign paroxysmal positional vertigo.* Journal of Clinical Neurology, 2010. **6**(2): p. 51-63.

122. Piza, M., *Meniere's disease: overview, epidemiology, and natural history.* Otolaryngologic Clinics of North America, 2002. **35**(3): p. 455-495.

123. Neff, B.A., et al., *Auditory and vestibular symptoms and chronic subjective dizziness in patients with Meniere's disease, vestibular migraine, and Meniere's disease with concomitant vestibular migraine.* Otology & Neurotology, 2012. **33**(7): p. 1235-1244.

124. Reploeg, M.D. and J.A. Goebel, *Migraine-associated dizziness: patient characteristics and management options.* Otology & neurotology, 2002. **23**(3): p. 364-371.

125. Fotuhi, M., et al., *Vestibular migraine: a critical review of treatment trials.* Journal of neurology, 2009. **256**(5): p. 711-716.

126. Barbosa, F. and T.R. Villa, *Vestibular migraine: diagnosis challenges and need for targeted treatment.* Arquivos de neuro-psiquiatria, 2016. **74**(5): p. 416-422.

127. Mullally, W.J., K. Hall, and R. Goldstein, *Efficacy of biofeedback in the treatment of migraine and tension type headaches.* Pain Physician, 2009. **12**(6): p. 1005-1011.

128. Neuhauser, H., et al., *Zolmitriptan for treatment of migrainous vertigo: a pilot randomized placebo-controlled trial.* Neurology, 2003. **60**(5): p. 882-883.

129. Bikhazi, P., C. Jackson, and M. Ruckenstein, *Efficacy of antimigrainous therapy in the treatment of migraine-associated dizziness.* The American journal of otology, 1997. **18**(3): p. 350-354.

130. Furman, J.M., D.A. Marcus, and C.D. Balaban, *Rizatriptan reduces vestibular-induced motion sickness in migraineurs.* The journal of headache and pain, 2011. **12**(1): p. 81.

131. Cassano, D., V. Pizza, and V. Busillo, *P074. Almotriptan in the acute treatment of Vestibular migraine: a retrospective study.* The journal of headache and pain, 2015. **16**(S1): p. A114.

132. Baloh, R.W., *Neurotology of migraine.* Headache: The Journal of Head and Face Pain, 1997. **37**(10): p. 615-621.

133. Çelebisoy, N., et al., *Acetazolamide in vestibular migraine prophylaxis: a retrospective study.* European Archives of Oto-Rhino-Laryngology, 2016. **273**(10): p. 2947-2951.

134. Taghdiri, F., et al., *Cinnarizine for the prophylaxis of migraine associated vertigo: a retrospective study.* SpringerPlus, 2014. **3**(1): p. 231.

135. Teggi, R., et al., *Fixed combination of cinnarizine and dimenhydrinate in the prophylactic therapy of vestibular migraine: an observational study.* Neurological Sciences, 2015. **36**(10): p. 1869-1873.

136. Lepcha, A., et al., *Flunarizine in the prophylaxis of migrainous vertigo: a randomized controlled trial.* European Archives of Oto-Rhino-Laryngology, 2014. **271**(11): p. 2931-2936.

137. Salmito, M.C., et al., *Prophylactic treatment of vestibular migraine.* Brazilian journal of otorhinolaryngology, 2017. **83**(4): p. 404-410.

138. Teive, H.A., et al., *Flunarizine and cinnarizine-induced parkinsonism: a historical and clinical analysis.* Parkinsonism & related disorders, 2004. **10**(4): p. 243-245.

139. Bisdorff, A.R., *Treatment of migraine related vertigo with lamotrigine an observational study.* Bull Soc Sci Med Grand Duche Luxemb, 2004. **2**: p. 103-108.

140. Morganti, L.O.G., et al., *Vestibular migraine: clinical and epidemiological aspects.* Brazilian journal of otorhinolaryngology, 2016. **82**(4): p. 397-402.

141. Gode, S., et al., *Clinical assessment of topiramate therapy in patients with migrainous vertigo.* Headache: The Journal of Head and Face Pain, 2010. **50**(1): p. 77-84.

142. Fernández, M.M., et al., *Pharmacological agents for the prevention of vestibular migraine.* Cochrane Database of Systematic Reviews, 2015(6).

143. Bisdorff, A.R., *Management of vestibular migraine.* Therapeutic advances in neurological disorders, 2011. **4**(3): p. 183-191.

144. Vitkovic, J., et al., *Vestibular rehabilitation outcomes in patients with and without vestibular migraine.* Journal of neurology, 2013. **260**(12): p. 3039-3048.

145. Whitney, S.L., et al., *Physical therapy for migraine-related vestibulopathy and vestibular dysfunction with history of migraine.* The Laryngoscope, 2000. **110**(9): p. 1528-1534.

146. Sticht, M.A., et al., *Endocannabinoid mechanisms influencing nausea,* in *International review of neurobiology.* 2015, Elsevier. p. 127-162.

147. Dieterich, M., M. Obermann, and N. Celebisoy, *Vestibular migraine: the most frequent entity of episodic vertigo.* Journal of neurology, 2016. **263**(1): p. 82-89.

148. Minor, L.B., D.A. Schessel, and J.P. Carey, *Meniere's disease.* Current opinion in neurology, 2004. **17**(1): p. 9-16.

149. Ishiyama, G., I. Lopez, and A. Ishiyama, *Aquaporins and Meniere's disease.* Current Opinion in Otolaryngology & Head and Neck Surgery, 2006. **14**(5): p. 332-336.

150. Rauch, S.D., *Clinical Hints and Precipitating Factors in Patients Suffering from Meniere's Disease.* Otolaryngologic Clinics of North America, 2010. **43**(5): p. 1011-1017.

151. Kangasniemi, E. and E. Hietikko, *The theory of autoimmunity in Meniere's disease is lacking evidence.* Auris Nasus Larynx, 2018. **45**(3): p. 399-406.

152. Vrabec, J.T., *Herpes simplex virus and Meniere's Disease.* The Laryngoscope, 2003. **113**(9): p. 1431-1438.

153. Bjorne, A., A. Berven, and G. Agerberg, *Cervical Signs and Symptoms in Patients with Meniere's Disease: A Controlled Study.* CRANIO®, 1998. **16**(3): p. 194-202.

154. Söderman, A.C.H., et al., *Stress as a Trigger of Attacks in Menière's Disease. A Case-Crossover Study.* The Laryngoscope, 2004. **114**(10): p. 1843-1848.

155. Nikolopoulos, T.P., et al., *Acoustic Neuroma Growth: A Systematic Review of the Evidence.* Otology & Neurotology, 2010. **31**(3): p. 478-485.

156. McLaughlin, E.J., et al., *Quality of Life in Acoustic Neuroma Patients.* Otology & Neurotology, 2015. **36**(4): p. 653-656.

157. Rosahl, S., et al., *Diagnostics and therapy of vestibular schwannomas–an interdisciplinary challenge.* GMS current topics in otorhinolaryngology, head and neck surgery, 2017. **16**.

158. McClelland, S.I., et al., *Impact of Race and Insurance Status on Surgical Approach for Cervical Spondylotic Myelopathy in the United States: A Population-Based Analysis.* Spine, 2017. **42**(3): p. 186-194.

159. Fusco, M.R., et al., *Current practices in vestibular schwannoma management: A survey of American and Canadian neurosurgeons.* Clinical Neurology and Neurosurgery, 2014. **127**: p. 143-148.

160. Hanley, K., *Symptoms of vertigo in general practice: a prospective study of diagnosis.* Br J Gen Pract, 2002. **52**(483): p. 809-812.

161. Wipperman, J., *Dizziness and vertigo.* Primary Care: Clinics in Office Practice, 2014. **41**(1): p. 115-131.

162. Bhattacharyya, N., et al., *Clinical practice guideline: benign paroxysmal positional vertigo.* Otolaryngology--Head and Neck Surgery, 2008. **139**(5_suppl): p. 47-81.

163. Schuknecht, H.F. and K. Kitamura, *Vestibular neuritis.* Annals of Otology, Rhinology & Laryngology, 1981. **90**(1_suppl): p. 1-19.

164. Perols, J.B., Olle, *Vestibular neuritis: a follow-up study.* Acta oto-laryngologica, 1999. **119**(8): p. 895-899.

165. Neuhauser, H.K. and T. Lempert. *Vertigo: epidemiologic aspects.* in *Seminars in neurology.* 2009. © Thieme Medical Publishers.

166. Baloh, R.W. and V. Honrubia, *Clinical neurophysiology of the vestibular system.* 2001: Oxford University Press, USA.

167. Hillier, S.L. and M. McDonnell, *Vestibular rehabilitation for unilateral peripheral vestibular dysfunction.* The Cochrane Library, 2011.

168. Brain Injury Research Institute. *What is a concussion?* ; Available from: http://www.protectthebrain.org/.

169. Centers for Disease Control and Prevention, *Traumatic Brain Injury and Concussion.* 2019.

170. Broglio, S.P., et al., *National Athletic Trainers' Association position statement: management of sport concussion.* Journal of athletic training, 2014. **49**(2): p. 245-265.

171. Eckhardt-Henn, A. and M. Dieterich, *Psychiatric disorders in otoneurology patients.* Neurologic clinics, 2005. **23**(3): p. 731-749.

172. Yuan, Q., et al., *Anxiety and depression among patients with different types of vestibular peripheral vertigo.* Medicine, 2015. **94**(5).

Image Credits

Image 1.1: shutterstock.com/Medical Art Inc

Image 1.2: shutterstock.com/ilusmedical

Image 1.3: shutterstock.com/maxcreatnz

Image 1.4: shutterstock.com/Designua

Front Cover Image: shutterstock.com/MDGRPHCS

Check out these other books by Mark Knoblauch

Challenge the Hand You Were Dealt: Strategies to battle back against adversity and improve your chances for success

Essentials of Writing and Publishing Your Self-Help Book

Living Low Sodium: A guide for understanding our relationship with sodium and how to be successful in adhering to a low-sodium diet

Outlining Tinnitus: A comprehensive guide to help you break free of the ringing in your ears

Overcoming Meniere's: How changing your lifestyle can change your life

Professional Writing in Kinesiology and Sports Medicine

Seven Ways To Make Running Not Suck

The Art of Efficiency: A guide for improving task management in the home to help maximize your leisure time

Understanding BPPV: Outlining the causes and effects of Benign Paroxysmal Positional Vertigo

About the Author

Mark is a small-town Kansas native who now lives in a suburb of Houston with his wife and two young daughters. His background is in the area of sports medicine, obtaining his bachelor's degree from Wichita State and his master's degree from the University of Nevada, Las Vegas. After working clinically as an athletic trainer for eight years, Mark returned to graduate school where he received his doctorate in Kinesiology from the University of Houston, followed by a postdoctoral assistantship in Molecular Physiology and Biophysics at Baylor College of Medicine in Houston, TX. He has been employed as a college professor at the University of Houston since 2013.

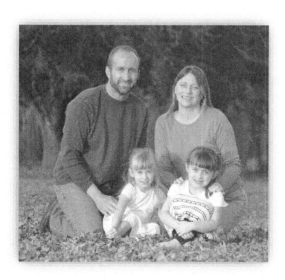

Made in United States
Orlando, FL
09 February 2023

29733468R00104